Ketamine for Depression

Ketamine for Depression

Dr. Stephen J. Hyde

Library of Congress Control Number: 2015913931
ISBN: Hardcover   978-1-5035-0955-9
                 Softcover   978-1-5035-0954-2
                 eBook   978-1-5035-0953-5

Print information available on the last page.

Cover image:
"Ketamine dropped on Photonegative, enlarged"
Sarah Ancelle Schoenfeld

Rev. date: 12/03/2018

To order additional copies of this book, contact:
Xlibris
1-800-455-039
www.Xlibris.com.au
Orders@Xlibris.com.au
719781

Contents

Appendices

Dedication

For my patients and for all who battle with depression and those who support them.

Acknowledgements

To the Xlibris family Carl, Ann, Marie, Mark and Stephanie for their expert advice and assistance.

To the ketamine doctors, Angelo, Varun, Graham and Diogo who have been so generous with their time and knowledge.

And thanks to my family for all their support, to my peer group for their patience, to Shelagh for her tolerance and for turning my bullet points into something readable, to the trail-blazing researchers and practitioners of ketamine and most of all to my patients whose stubbornness and courage have encouraged me to continue to look for better treatments.

Foreword

"Truth is indeed stranger than fiction! Many years ago when I was a clinical pharmacologist-working part time at the Lafayette Clinic, I ran the drug abuse-screening laboratory. I was often referred drug abuse patients by the attending psychiatrists. Several referrals dealt with phencyclidine and ketamine drug abuse, especially in the late '70s and early '80s. A number of these patients were mentally depressed, taking various antidepressants off and on. I remember one young lady, in particular, who was a chronic phencyclidine and later ketamine abuser. She had serious bouts of mental depression. I asked her why she took these illicit drugs rather than her usual antidepressant medications. Her answer was "Oh, doctor, my antidepressants don't work as well." She stated that ketamine and phencyclidine worked quickly and were much better antidepressants but they didn't last as long so she took them again and again. I promptly recommended that she stop this bizarre practice because it would only harm her. I never pursued the possible antidepressant actions of ketamine. After all - I knew better! ...

.... When Zarate et al. in 2006 reported their positive results with ketamine in a randomised trial of treatment-resistant major depression, I became a believer. I thought of my Lafayette Clinic referral patient of years ago. Again I learned an important lesson. Doctor, listen to your patients and what they tell you!"

Edward F Domino MD who, in 1964, was the first doctor to administer Ketamine to a human.
("Taming the Ketamine Tiger."
Anesthesiology, V 113 • No 3 • September 2010)

Chapter 1

My Journey with Ketamine

I work as a psychiatrist in private practice, seeing people who are not quite ill enough to need to be in hospital but not quite well enough to be managed solely in general practice. Although I am now semi-retired, I still see nearly 90 long-term patients who have made it quite clear to me that I need to stay around until they are cured.

This is proving to be difficult.

I had been vaguely aware of ketamine from sporadic reports of its use over the past 18 years, but what really attracted my attention was what happened 6 years ago when one of my patients was given a 10-day subcutaneous (under the skin) ketamine infusion for severe persistent pain. This treatment worked well for her pain, but it also noticeably improved the severe depressive symptoms she was experiencing at that time. Was it a coincidence? Perhaps not having the pain had made the difference. My interest subsided.

In early 2014, I was trying to help a man with chronic, severe obsessive-compulsive disorder (OCD) who needed six hours to complete his bathroom rituals, and we were discussing the possibility of brain surgery. One must bear in mind that brain surgery is reserved for the most intractable of cases; all possible treatments have to have been tried and failed before surgery is contemplated.

I then read that intravenous ketamine had been helpful in reducing OCD symptoms in a small group of patients treated in America. I discussed this with my patient, and as he was keen to try anything that could help, I sought permission from our local private hospital to test this treatment. The process of obtaining and submitting the required information to be reviewed by the Medical Advisory Committee was time consuming, and there was then a period of two months to wait before the next meeting of the committee. During this time, I explored all the research I could find on ketamine, downloading over 500 studies and articles from the fields of anaesthetics, pain medicine, and psychiatry.

Deep into this process and deeper still into Google I found two articles which led me to change my way of thinking dramatically.

The first was by a group of Brazilian psychiatrists, Diogo Lara and colleagues,[1] who reported success in helping people with treatment-resistant mood disorders using very-low-dose sublingual (placed under the tongue) ketamine. This approach was in stark contrast to the vast majority of published trials to date, which have used the intravenous route, requiring hospitals, anaesthetists, intensive monitoring, and not the least, considerable expense.

This led me to consider the next big question: how safe is it to take ketamine for extended periods? Most of the early trials had involved either the use of single doses or, at most, treatment for two weeks. However, the second article I discovered described the quite remarkable work of Varun Jaitly,[2] an anaesthetist and pain medicine specialist working in the United Kingdom. He had been using sublingual ketamine over the past 15 years to treat a variety of chronic pain conditions not responding to the usual remedies. He reported that ketamine was helpful in around 20% of these very-tough-to-treat conditions, but more importantly, he had monitored patients over the years and had not observed major problems with long-term use (one patient has been taking it 3 times a day for 15 years). In particular, there had been no signs of dependence or addiction nor any indications of bladder problems that can affect those who abuse ketamine by taking very high doses regularly for non-medical reasons.

Encouraged by these reports and by other small-scale studies, I found describing the use of oral ketamine I developed a treatment protocol, and after discussions with my peer review group, I began treating some of my most difficult patients with the low-dose sublingual method in November 2014 (see the appendices for the treatment process, consent form, sample scripts, and patient information sheets).

The most notable features of my treatment are:

1. After a trial dose of ketamine monitored in my consulting rooms, patients self-administer further doses at home, taking it every second day initially. They continue with their current treatments.
2. If there is no improvement, the dose is gradually increased until either clear benefit has been obtained or side effects become troublesome.
3. Those who improve fully then extend the interval between their doses by only taking another when there are signs that their mood is slipping. At this point, trials of reducing other medications can begin.
4. For those who partially improve, we continue to test combinations of talking therapies, medications, dietary change, and exercise along with ketamine to try to get the best response. Ketamine may be stopped for a trial period to clarify its benefits.
5. For those who do not respond, we continue to search for better treatments.

Usually, I would expect with any new treatment, be it medication or a different psychological approach (e.g. mindfulness therapy), that around 10% of the hard-to-treat patients will obtain an appreciable benefit. However, since starting ketamine, about 70% of patients in my trial have clearly improved, and 40% have now made full recoveries. Some have not needed to take ketamine for months. This mirrors the results from trials using the intravenous, intramuscular, subcutaneous, intranasal, and oral routes of administration.

From my experience, there are major advantages to the low-dose sublingual method over these other approaches.

1. Patients require less ketamine over the course of treatment due to the lower doses being administered.
2. Side effects are minimal at these dosage levels.
3. It is very much more affordable for both patients and the government if people can take their ketamine at home.
4. More people can be seen and treated compared with time-consuming clinic and hospital systems.

There are also some possible disadvantages:

1. This could encourage the quick-fix magic-bullet approach: 'Just take this and all will be well.'
2. There is a higher potential for misuse. To prevent this from occurring, good patient selection is required together with close follow-up for those who may be at risk (e.g. people who have experienced dependence or addiction to other agents).
3. The low starting dose and the slow-building titration means that for most it will take a week before some response is evident and two to three weeks for a marked improvement. For some, this will be too long, and hospital-based intravenous ketamine and intensive support may be required.

While there are no easy answers to the complex and difficult situations that some people endure, my experience has been that ketamine combined with counselling can give people the ability to make quite startling changes to their usual ways of dealing with their problems.

This is RJ's story.

> I have battled severe depression and anxiety for many years.
>
> Eleven years ago, I had to leave my job, where I worked in aged care, and I was put on the disability support pension for my depression and anxiety. Over the years, with Dr Hyde's help, I have tried many medications, and I have had quite extensive electroconvulsive therapy (ECT).
>
> Last year, Dr Hyde spoke to me about ketamine. After many discussions, we decided it was in my best interest to try this medication. I started on a very low dose, which I put under my tongue for four minutes, and I administered the medication every four to five days.
>
> I have had regular visits with Dr Hyde so he could check my progress and alter the dose and the timeframe as needed. The only side effect that I have when I take my medication is I feel a little sleepy, but that is okay as I take it at bedtime.

Almost instantaneously, I noticed the difference in myself. I became more alert. I felt happiness that I had not felt for years. I have so much more energy. I no longer want to sleep my life away, and most importantly, I want to live. I enjoy my life so much more now.

In January 2015, I did something I never thought I would be able to do. I enrolled in college to do a diploma in community services (case management course). I am doing really well in the course, and I am enjoying my studies and time spent with my classmates. After I graduate, I am hoping to further my studies and eventually become a youth worker.

I honestly can say I never in my wildest dreams thought I would be doing this and thinking along the lines of re-entering the workforce. I never thought that, after all these years, I could accomplish this.

I truly believe with all my heart that ketamine has totally changed my life. I wish it had been available to me years ago.

Life is good, and I can truly say ketamine is this girl's best friend.

Here is an account from another of my patients who tried ketamine

Hi, my name is Gavin. I have suffered with depression for about 20 years and I've have tried lots of different things to help me with my depression - ECT, so many different pills I can't remember, alpha-stim, acupuncture, diets. At one stage I spent a year in bed to stay away from life and took many different pills which gave me some relief but they had side effects for me some which are too hard to talk about.

I am on a new drug now, ketamine and it's been a life changer for me. I started on 10mg and it helped for about 4 days, the dose went up gradually and the times I needed to take it got further apart. I'm now on 100mg, which I think is good for me. I've been on it for some months now and it's lasting longer and longer, more than a month now between doses. These days I take notice of what gets me down - if there is a reason for it, if there is shit in life that does it, I don't take ketamine. But, if I am down on the second day I take it then and the next day I'm fine.

My doctor told me not to drink beer on the day when taking it, but I did and I am telling you - don't!

I don't like to recommend things but I'm so glad I got the chance to try it; I never want to go without it again. The people around me tell me this is the best I have been in 15 years. Gavin

So my journey began, but before proceeding further, I'll take you back to the very beginning, the birth of the ketamine story.

References

1. Diogo R. Lara, Luisa W. Bisol, and Luciano R. Munari, 'Antidepressant, Mood Stabilizing and Procognitive Effects of Very Low Dose Sublingual Ketamine in Refractory Unipolar and Bipolar Depression', *International Journal of Neuropsychopharmacology*, 16 (2013), 2111–2117. DOI:10.1017/S1461145713000485.
2. V. K. Jaitly, 'Sublingual Ketamine in Chronic Pain: Service Evaluation by Examining More Than 200 Patient Years of Data', *Journal of Observational Pain Medicine*, 1/2 (2013).

Chapter 2

A Short History of Ketamine

Ketamine was first synthesised in 1962 at the Parke Davis Laboratories in Michigan by Calvin Stevens, a professor of organic chemistry at Wayne State University, Detroit. This new drug was a derivative of phencyclidine (angel dust), which was first made in 1956 and trialled as an anaesthetic. It was effective, but it had too many unwanted side effects, including prolonged bizarre hallucinations, so the decision was made to look for alternatives.

Ketamine (then known as CI-581) progressed through animal studies and was first administered to a human, a volunteer from the Jackson Prison in Michigan, on 3 August 1964 by Edward F. Domino, a professor of pharmacology, and Guenter Corssen, a professor of anaesthesiology.

Edward recalls:

> Guenter and I gradually increased the dose from no effect, to conscious but 'spaced out,' and finally to enough for general anaesthesia. Our findings were remarkable! The overall incidence of side effects was about one out of three volunteers. Frank emergence delirium was minimal. Most of our subjects described strange experiences like a feeling of floating in outer space and having no feeling in their arms or legs.
>
> In discussing the unusual actions of ketamine with my wife, Toni, I mentioned that the subjects were 'disconnected'

from their environment. Toni came up with the term 'dissociative anaesthetic.' That is what ketamine is still called today.[1]

After further trials, ketamine was approved in 1970 by the Food and Drug Administration authority as an anaesthetic suitable for use in children, adults, and the elderly. Specifically, the indications for use were for diagnostic and surgical procedures not requiring muscle relaxation, for induction of anaesthesia prior to the administration of other general anaesthetic agents, and for supplementing low-potency agents (e.g. nitrous oxide).

Unlike many other anaesthetics, it did not significantly slow breathing or lower blood pressure, thus making it a very safe agent to use particularly in settings where intensive support and monitoring were not available. These qualities led to it being used as a 'buddy drug' for American soldiers in the Vietnam War. Each soldier would carry a vial of ketamine that could be injected intramuscularly into a wounded comrade, providing pain relief and a degree of sedation. It was considered to be safer than using opiates in that setting, and its military use continues today.

'Ketamine has become a recommended analgesic agent in the combat environment in Afghanistan due to its safety profile, favourable hemodynamic characteristics in severely injured combat casualties, rapid onset and ease of use. Current Tactical Combat Casualty Care guidelines allow for its use even in the setting of eye trauma and head injuries in which the person is conscious enough to demonstrate the need for analgesia. A recent study evaluating the use of analgesic agents at the point-of-injury found no adverse events from the use of ketamine— even under the harshest conditions with minimal to no monitoring. It is a recommended agent by the Wilderness Medical Society for use in remote environments. Even in the hands of non-physician practitioners it appears safe.'[2]

Ketamine is also currently used by the Royal Flying Doctor Service in Australia for sedation during air transport and is regarded as an effective and safer alternative to the use of general anaesthesia and intubation.[3]

All medicines we humans benefit from have at some stage been tested on animals. Their use in research does not always meet with universal approval, but one of the great benefits is that agents tested and approved are then also available to treat animal disorders.

As stated by the Federation of Veterinarians of Europe in 2015: 'Ketamine is very widely used for anaesthesia and analgesia by the veterinary profession. It is an essential anaesthetic for veterinary use because it is the only injectable anaesthetic that is safe and well tested in the full range of species that the veterinarian must treat. This includes both large and small domestic animals, children's pets and laboratory animals, large, wild and zoo animals as well as birds and reptiles. It is safely used by virtually every veterinary practice throughout Europe and the rest of the world.'

In the 1970s, ketamine—colloquially known as Special K, Kit Kat, or Vitamin K—began to seep into the counterculture along with lysergic acid diethylamide (LSD) and other psychedelic agents that were being tried at the time. This was the era of the 'psychonauts', most notably John Lilly and Marcia Moore; both are dedicated explorers of inner space who wrote detailed accounts of their self-experiments. I'll explore more about their adventures in chapter 6.

Ketamine was also used as one of the therapeutic agents in psychedelic psychotherapy until the alarm was raised concerning the perceived hazards of LSD (acid) and psilocybin (magic mushrooms) in particular. Laws were passed, effectively banning their use in the early seventies, and ketamine was the only agent in this group to remain a legal drug. It has only been in recent years that interest has revived, and small studies are now being conducted into the use of LSD, MDMA and other psychedelic agents in psychiatry.

In Russia E. M. Krupitsky and colleagues used ketamine to supplement their usual treatments for alcoholism. They reported in 1997 that 65% of patients receiving both ketamine and standard treatment improved compared to 25% with the standard treatment alone.

They commented, 'The studies of the underlying psychological mechanisms have indicated that ketamine-assisted psychedelic therapy of alcoholic patients induces a harmonisation of the Minnesota Multiphasic Personality Inventory (MMPI) personality profile, positive transformation of nonverbalized (mostly unconscious) self-concept and emotional attitudes to various aspects of self and other people, positive changes in life values and purposes, important insights into the meaning of life and an increase in the level of spiritual development. Most importantly, these psychological changes were shown to favour a sober lifestyle.[4]

Ketamine became part of the rave drug party scene in the 1990s with the euphoria and heightened sensory awareness it induced being attractive to partygoers. Its use has since fluctuated according to availability, cost, and culture. In 2014 an Australian study reported that 1.7% of those aged 14 and over had reported using ketamine in their lifetimes, 0.3% in the past year.[5] In the USA, the 2011 Monitoring the Future survey reported that 1.7% of twelfth graders had tried ketamine, a reduction from the 2000 figure of 2.5%. Use in other places is higher, particularly in Hong Kong, where nearly 50% of users of illicit drugs describe it as their drug of choice.

It is interesting that in 2015 China, as part of a campaign to limit the illicit use of ketamine in Hong Kong, applied to the United Nations for ketamine to be reclassified, potentially severely limiting its use around the world. This aroused strong opposition globally as it remains the most widely used anaesthetic in the Third World because of its safety profile. Fears were expressed that the reclassification would cause severe restrictions in its availability and use. China, to the relief of many, has withdrawn its application. Ketamine remains on the World Health Organisation's list of essential medicines, meaning that it should be stocked by every hospital.

In the psychiatric field during the 1990s, John H. Krystal and his colleagues at the Yale University School of Medicine were studying the drug as a way of understanding schizophrenia. Ketamine is classed as a dissociative drug because it produces feelings of disconnection from one's self and reality, which are similar to some of the symptoms of schizophrenia; very high doses elicit complete depersonalisation and profoundly altered perception. Some have described this 'k-hole' as similar to an out-of-body experience.[6]

Its use was also explored for the treatment of eating disorders. In 1998 Professor I. H. Mills and colleagues from University of Cambridge published a fascinating account of their treatment of 15 patients suffering from severe treatment-refractory eating disorders.[7] They gave their patients continuous infusions of intravenous ketamine at the sub-anaesthetic dose of 20 mg/hour for ten hours. They also gave an opiate antagonist to reduce both sedation and the risk of hallucinations.

Nine of the 15 responded with prolonged remissions after receiving between two and nine infusions. These were given at intervals of five days to three weeks according to clinical response. The remaining six did not respond despite being given a minimum of five treatments.

For this group of patients, who are notoriously difficult to treat, this was a stunning result. The side effect burden was low, with headaches and nausea apparent early on, and there were only two reports of hallucinations that Professor Mills attributed to giving the ketamine too quickly on one occasion and giving an insufficient dose of the opiate antagonist on the other.

The following is a summary of one the responders:

> Patient 8 suffered from the relatively rare condition of compulsive thirsting. She would cut her fluid intake to extremely low levels and on rare occasions had gone for a week or more with zero fluid intake. Previously she had had anorexia nervosa with short phases of bulimia. Compulsive thirsting was always associated with a sharp fall in food intake. After four ketamine treatments she drank normally and her compulsion and depression scores fell sharply. After discharge, she returned to a demanding job and relapsed. A short stay in hospital with two ketamine treatments restored normal eating and drinking. A month later while she was an outpatient she had a slight relapse and was given one further ketamine treatment. She then drank enough fluid each day to remain out of hospital while being followed for the next 7 months.

Interest had also grown in ketamine's pain-relieving qualities, and from the mid nineties, trials were begun in patients with severe chronic pain conditions not responding to the standard remedies. Neurologist Robert Schwartzman of Drexel University College of Medicine in Philadelphia and colleagues at the University of Tübingen in Germany used ketamine to treat 41 patients with reflex sympathetic dystrophy (RSD). This is a rare, disabling pain disorder in which ordinary sensations—such as touch, warmth, and coolness—are perceived as painful and minor knocks are agonising. RSD is associated with nerve injuries after accidents or surgery, for example.

After five-day continuous intravenous infusions, 14 of the 41 experienced relief lasting for months for some, an outstanding result in this group. He also collaborated with a group in Mexico, but some major complications and one fatality have impeded the widespread application of this approach. More-modest regimes, some using intramuscular and subcutaneous routes, were also helpful and continue to be used for a range of difficult-to-treat pain conditions.

Some pain physicians, notably Godfrey Batchelor and later Varun Jaitly in the UK, seeking simpler, more-accessible treatment began using sublingual ketamine at relatively low doses for chronic pain conditions, and Jaitly continues to do so to this day in his pain clinic at the Royal Albert Edward Infirmary in Wigan. I've described his groundbreaking work more fully in chapter 7, 'The Ketamine Doctors'.[8]

And as for depression, in the next chapter, I will outline the research that began in 2000 into the use of ketamine for treatment of this illness.

References

1. Edward F. Domino, 'Taming the Ketamine Tiger', *Anesthesiology* (2010).
2. S. Schauer et al., *Emergency Physicians Monthly* (April 2015).
3. Minh Le Cong et al., *Emergency Medical Journal* [online journal] (May 2011).
4. E. M. Krupitsky et al., *Journal of Psychoactive Drugs* (April 1997).
5. Australian Institute of Health and Wellbeing 2014.
6. Maia Szalavitz, 'Tackling Depression with Ketamine', *New Scientist* (January 2007).
7. I. H. Mills, G. R. Park, A. R. Manara, R. J. Merriman, 'Treatment of Compulsive Behaviour in Eating Disorders with Intermittent Ketamine Infusions', *QJM*, 91/7 (July 1998), 493–503.
8. V. K. Jaitly, 'Sublingual Ketamine in Chronic Pain: Service Evaluation by Examining More Than 200 Patient Years of Data', *Journal of Observational Pain Medicine*, 1/2 (2013).

Chapter 3

History of Ketamine
Treatment for Depression

In this chapter, I will explore the research conducted so far into the use of ketamine for the treatment of depression. The articles to be discussed cover the time from 2000 to 2018 and have been published in reputable journals. I have not reviewed every study as some just confirm previous work without breaking new ground, but the bulk of the published work is discussed here. Some of the single-case reports are particularly interesting as they indicate ideas and leads for more detailed work in the future. I have provided general summaries of the studies, but for those interested in the in-depth details, there is a full reference section at the end of this chapter.

Various factors are important when assessing the results of a research trial. These include the reputation and track record of the researchers, the number of subjects being assessed, and whether the study is being done in one or multiple centres.

In addition, because both subjects' and researchers' expectations can influence the outcome of studies, finding ways of limiting this bias, for example, by using placebos is most important.

For those unfamiliar with medical research terms, here are some you will find mentioned throughout this chapter:

- *double-blind*—Neither the investigator nor the subject knows who is receiving the active treatment or the inactive comparator.

- *randomised*—Subjects are allocated to receive the active or inactive treatment in a random fashion.
- *placebo-controlled*—All therapies have effects that arise from the expectations of the researchers and the subjects. Placebos (i.e. inert or inactive therapies) are used to try to discriminate between the wished-for result and the result actually due to the active treatment being studied.
- *crossover*—Subjects are given one treatment, and then after an interval after which it is expected that any possible effect of that treatment has subsided, a second treatment is given.
- *response*—This is usually defined as a 50% reduction in the intensity of the symptoms which were experienced before the commencement of the trial.
- *remission*—This is a strong response often given as a cut-off point on rating scales. It is important to note that even patients in remission may experience some symptoms. Someone who is fully recovered would be seen as being asymptomatic.
- *racemic ketamine*—This is the most common form made for use. It is a mixture of R- and S-ketamine. S-ketamine is sometimes used in Europe. Unless specified, any references to ketamine indicate the racemic compound.
- *psychomimetic effects*—These are the experiences of depersonalisation (a person feeling unreal), derealisation (the world looking strange), and hallucinations that can occur particularly with higher doses and rapid administration of ketamine.
- *treatment-resistant depression*—Varying definitions exist which could account for some of the variations in trial results. There needs to be a lack of response to at least two adequate trials of antidepressants for the current depressive episode before the term *treatment-resistant* is applied. In many cases, patients have also failed to respond to psychotherapy and ECT.
- *open-label ketamine*—Both giver and receiver know the treatment is ketamine. This is the situation in most of the case reports and observational studies.
- *depression*—This is an illness characterised by prolonged episodes of low mood and associated symptoms, including anhedonia (lack of feelings of pleasure), problems with thinking and concentration, sleep and appetite disturbance, and for some, suicidal thoughts.

- *unipolar depression*—The patient suffers from depressive episodes only.
- *bipolar depression*—The patient experiences sustained episodes of elevated mood as well as depressive episodes (previously known as manic depression).
- *The N-methyl-D-aspartate (NMDA) receptor*—Present in over 80% of the brain's neurones, this is the 'docking centre' where ketamine binds and affects the function of electrochemical pathways.
- *electroconvulsive therapy (ECT)*—This is the fastest-acting and most effective treatment for severe depression available over the past 75 years. However, some responders relapse quickly, and some have problems with memory loss, particularly in the first month following a course of treatment.

As Maia Szalavitz said in her 2007 article in the *New Scientist*: 'The possibility that Ketamine could lift depression was first mooted in the late 1990s, when Krystal and his colleagues at Yale were studying the drug as a way of understanding schizophrenia. Ketamine is classed as a "dissociative" because it produces feelings of disconnection from one's self and reality which are similar to some of the symptoms of schizophrenia; very high doses elicit complete depersonalisation and profoundly altered perception.

In the course of his work, Krystal had come across case reports from the 1950s and 1960s suggesting that depressed tuberculosis patients given the tuberculosis drug d-cycloserine, which has pharmacological similarities to ketamine, sometimes reported rapid release from their depression. He also found research showing that some existing antidepressants worked in a similar way.'[1]

Robert Berman and Krystal's group put two and two together and began a trial using ketamine, the results of which were published in 2000 and still resonate today. This study was a randomised, placebo-controlled, double-blind trial with a crossover after one week.[2]

They recruited eight medication-free patients with treatment-resistant depression and gave each of them an infusion of ketamine or a placebo (saline). A week later, the subjects were 'crossed over' so those who had received ketamine then received the placebo and vice versa. The group had experience with using intravenous ketamine from their previous studies and used 0.5 mg/kg of body weight, which was a quarter of the standard anaesthetic dose. (Interestingly, there is some evidence that some standard antidepressants work more quickly given intravenously, but this has never become established practice.)

Ketamine Produces Rapid Antidepressant Effects

- **NMDA receptor antagonist and dissociative anesthetic at hi doses.**
- **At low doses,** ketamine produces a rapid response in treatment resistant **depressed patients**

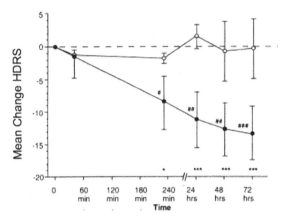

Berman, Heninger, Charney, Krystal, and colleagues 2000

Image courtesy of Ronald Duman

Four of the eight patients had a response (a 50% reduction in symptoms) during the three-day follow-up period. One of the eight responded to the saline infusion. All symptoms had returned to baseline in one to two weeks. All patients reported improved mood during the 40-minute infusion. Overall, the results were impressive in this very-hard-to-treat group. The main lessons to emerge from this study were that ketamine could work in people who had not been helped by the currently available treatments. Side effects did occur, with euphoria and perceptual changes being described, but these were transient and tolerable. Ketamine worked quickly, and the effects of a single dose of ketamine would last about a week for responders. Conversely, standard antidepressants typically take several weeks to bring about some improvement and six to eight weeks to achieve full recovery in only a third of users.

In addition, as the researchers later pointed out, the volunteers did not feel better because they were on a high similar to a cocaine buzz, which some depressed people used to lift their mood. 'I would really contrast ketamine's effects on depression to those of cocaine,' says Krystal. 'The hallmark of drugs of abuse is a transient euphoria followed by persistent dysphoria—the cocaine crash. Ketamine is fundamentally different. There may be brief euphoric effects but when those symptoms go away, instead of being dysphoric or hung-over, what we saw was remarkable.'

So ketamine was effective, and there was rapid improvement and tolerable side effects. What could go wrong?

The results were published in a reputable journal to a resounding silence. Ketamine abuse and addiction had been a growing concern for the authorities, leading to its further restriction in 1999 in the USA as a Schedule III non-narcotic substance under the Controlled Substances Act. As a result, it was even more of a taboo drug, hardly likely to be taken seriously for therapy. In addition, as ketamine had long been off-patent, there was no incentive for pharmaceutical companies to further this line of research.

The next published work was from A. Kudoh and colleagues at the Department of Anesthesiology, Hakodate Watanabe Hospital, Aomori, Japan, in 2002.[3] They had noted that patients with depression reported more post-operative pain and wondered whether using ketamine as one of the anaesthetic agents would have an effect on both post-operative depression and pain levels.

They reported from a study in patients undergoing orthopaedic surgery, where 70 patients suffering from current depressive illness were randomly split into 2 groups. The first group was given ketamine as an anaesthetic at 1.0 mg/kg of body weight along with other standard anaesthetic agents; the second group received the standard agents only. A non-depressed control group was also given ketamine. The ketamine group had significantly lower depression and pain scores one day after surgery, and the difference had disappeared by three days post-operatively.

Their results indicated that ketamine had both significant pain-relieving and antidepressant activity, and notably, there was no difference in the side effects experienced by either group. They had used a higher dose of ketamine than the Berman study, and the ketamine was added to the patients' usual medication for depression, whereas in the Berman study, patients had been medication-free.

One would have thought that this result published in a reputable journal and demonstrating such positive results would have led to, at the very least, a replication study and an increased use of ketamine in this situation; after all, we know people with pain and depression recover more slowly from any procedure. This did not happen.

In 2005 Robert Ostroff and colleagues, in a letter to the editor of the American Journal of Psychiatry,[4] described the case of a 47-year-old woman with severe treatment-resistant depression who was referred for electroconvulsive therapy (ECT) shortly after ceasing anti-epileptic medication. She was given ketamine at 0.5 mg/kg as part of the anaesthesia for the first ECT, but she failed to have a convulsion (an adequate convulsion is necessary for effective ECT). However, she reported on waking from the procedure feeling an immediate improvement in mood and appetite.

Two days later, she had another ECT with ketamine again being used as an induction agent, but once again she did not have a seizure. Despite this, she reported a further improvement in mood and now rated herself as being 7/10 (10 being her usual self) as opposed to her 2/10 rating prior to the first ECT. Two days later, her mood again began to decline, and she was subsequently given four more treatments, all with full seizures being obtained, before fully recovering.

It would appear highly likely that ketamine had caused the rapid short-lived improvement in mood described after the two failed ECTs. There have since been a number of studies using ketamine as anaesthesia for ECT as a way of potentially reducing the memory problems some experience in the short term following ECT. Although no clear benefit has emerged from this work, one recent study of ketamine compared directly with ECT showed that repeated intravenous ketamine worked more quickly than ECT over a two-week period.[5]

The next published study emanated from Australia in 2006. Graeme Correll, an anaesthetist, and Graham Futter, a psychiatrist, who both worked at the Mackay Base Hospital in Queensland, described the effect of ketamine treatment on two patients with depression. Interestingly, their regime involved the use of a continuous intravenous infusion of ketamine over five days. They had noted that patients given a similar infusion for CRPS (chronic regional pain syndrome), a severe chronic pain disorder, who had coexisting depression experienced significant lifts in mood when their pain was treated. They then decided to apply the pain protocols to see if they would work in pure depression.

Their first patient had an 18-month history of depression unsuccessfully treated with the antidepressants citalopram, mirtazapine, venlafaxine, and then ECT.

> The ketamine was commenced at 15 mg/hr and titrated to 27.5 mg/hr. At this level, the patient was 'a bit heady' but did not hallucinate. Nursing staff and family noted a positive improvement in the patient after 24 hours, particularly a decrease in fluctuation of mood. After 48 hours she began to show an interest in her pastimes and after 72 hours began cooking meals and snacks for patients and staff. She was discharged after five days and continued to improve for several weeks. At a follow-up visit one month after treatment, her 9-year-old son said, 'I have got my mummy back.' Twelve months after her treatment, she continues to be a bright, happy person and is participating in a 'return to work' program. Her current medication is citalopram.

The second patient had a 16-year history of depression unsuccessfully treated with fluoxetine, nefazodone, mirtazapine, venlafaxine, amisulpride, lithium, and ECT. He was given a five-day IV infusion of ketamine at 0.3 mg/kg/hr. His BDI (Beck Depression Inventory), a depression scale, improved from 52 to 9 in four days. He later relapsed twice after 2.5 months and then at 8.5 months and had two further five-day infusions, which were successful.[5]

Although this method is impractical for large numbers of patients, this remains a very important study. Firstly, it confirmed Berman's finding that a rapid response to ketamine was possible in treatment-resistant patients.

Secondly, both patients showed long-term improvement with this 'saturation' approach. Thirdly, the second patient's relapses were effectively treated with the same procedure. The finding that relapses could occur after long intervals of wellness confirmed that ketamine is not a cure for most patients. This was the same conclusion pain physicians reached from their experience of treating CRPS, where relapses were common but patients responded well to repeated infusions.

To my knowledge, there have been no further reports of the use of continuous infusions. Just as with Mills's successful use in 1998 of ketamine infusions to treat eating disorders, there seemed no interest in replicating and extending this knowledge. If ketamine indeed is a viable alternative to ECT and you are a patient with severe depression, which would you prefer to try first?

At this point, six years after the groundbreaking Berman study, a replication attempt was finally made. Dennis Charney, who had taken part in the initial Berman trial, moved to the Bethesda National Institute of Mental Health (NIMH) and there teamed up with a group including Carlos Zarate.

This was a randomised, placebo-controlled, double-blind, crossover study of 18 patients with treatment-resistant major depression. Each was given a single intravenous infusion of ketamine 0.5 mg/kg over 40 minutes. As with Berman's study, no medications had been given in the previous two weeks.

The trial results were impressive. His team had recruited people who, on average, had failed to get relief from six different antidepressants; four had tried ECT, the treatment of last resort. Of the 17 who completed the trial, 12 experienced a strong antidepressant response within hours of receiving ketamine, and for six patients, the response lasted a week or more. As Zarate described, the improved patients reported that their depression 'lifted'.[6]

Larger Replication Study Demonstrating Rapid Antidepressant Actions of Ketamine

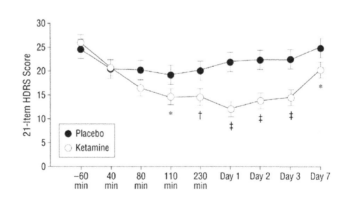

Zarate, Charney, et al., at NIMH et al., 2006

Image courtesy of Ronald Duman

'Zarate's results make all the difference,' Krystal commented. 'Replication is everything. One exciting finding is a footnote but a replication makes it much more interesting, particularly by a different group. It has opened up discussion about rapid-acting antidepressants.'

One might have expected that with this replication, there would have been a surge in interest in the use of ketamine, but unfortunately, progress remained slow and spasmodic.

Zarate's was another single-infusion study, and it indeed appeared to work for some in the short term, but so does a night without sleep for some with severe depression (at least until they sleep again). What was needed was work studying the effects of repeated infusions.

One step in this direction was made by Michael Liebrenz. His case report was published in 2007 in the *Swiss Medical Weekly*:

> A 55-year-old male subject with a treatment-resistant major depression and a co-occurring alcohol and benzodiazepine dependence received an intravenous infusion of 0.5 mg/kg ketamine over a period of 50 minutes.
>
> Over the previous five years the subject had been treated with a wide variety of antidepressants as well as intensive cognitive behavioural therapy. All the psychopharmacological and psychotherapeutic interventions were tolerated well, but failed to achieve remission.
>
> After the ketamine infusion, his BDI improved from 26 to 9 in two days. He remained well for 7 days before relapsing.[7]

Liebrenz later reported in 2009 that he had given another course of two successive infusions of ketamine to this patient. There had been a similar positive response to the first infusion and a lesser response to the second infusion in that the time to relapse was faster, being 7 days as opposed to 35 days following the first infusion.[8]

Liebrenz had shown that multiple infusions for patients were feasible and that it was also reasonable to expect a positive outcome even for a patient with current alcohol and benzodiazepine dependence.

The next published study was by G. Paslakis et al. from the Central Institute of Mental Health, Department of Psychiatry and Psychotherapy,

Mannheim, Germany. This appeared in 2009 and was notable for a number of reasons:

1. It was the first to report on the use of oral ketamine for the treatment of depression.
2. Paslakis used S-ketamine, the optical isomer, instead of the racemic mixture (R- and S-ketamine).
3. They observed that two patients with uncomplicated, albeit severe, depression responded, whereas two with prominent personality problems as well as depression did not.
4. Their oral dose was 1.25 mg/kg body weight dosage of ketamine. Taken orally, about 20% of the ketamine is available to the brain.
5. The ketamine was combined with the antidepressant venlafaxine, and both were started at the same time. The ketamine was continued for a further two weeks, and those who improved maintained their venlafaxine after the ketamine was ceased.
6. There were no problems with side effects, and the benefit was evident after one week. It would have been unusual for anyone taking venlafaxine alone to have improved at this point.

They reported: 'A 42-year-old dental technician was admitted for treatment of recurrent depressive disorder, presenting a severe episode with characteristic melancholic features. In this case, we were able to identify distinct causal factors related to the onset of depression approximately 18 months earlier. In order to experience some relief, the patient had begun to drink alcohol in an abusive, but not dependent manner. In this case treatment with 150 mg oral S-ketamine as add-on to 150 mg venlafaxine led to quick and substantial improvement of symptoms.'[9]

This was a small study, but some very interesting questions arose from it.

First is on their use of S-ketamine, which had been approved and used in Europe since 1998. Ketamine is a racemic mixture consisting of two components, R- and S-ketamine. In contrast to the usually prescribed ketamine mixture, S-ketamine is reported to be less prone to psychomimetic side effects, such as derealisation and hallucinations.

Currently, research is being conducted into using S-ketamine as an intranasal formulation.

Secondly, there was the use of oral ketamine instead of the previous intravenous route. This method is clearly more practical and economic if effective.

Starting ketamine in combination with a standard antidepressant is also an intriguing idea. It can be safely combined with most current antidepressants, and if it could provide the initial boost and then be stopped, more might respond overall. Also to consider is the dangerous two-week period after starting an antidepressant, during which there is a reported increase in suicidal thinking, particularly in the younger age groups. An earlier response would help greatly to reduce this risk.

Then again, would the same result have been obtained without the venlafaxine?

The 2009 study of ketamine by Price, Charney, Knock and Matthew,[10] showed a strong positive benefit from the use of ketamine, both in alleviating depressive symptoms and in reducing suicidal thoughts. However, actively suicidal patients were excluded from this trial.

Twenty-six patients had one infusion with an 80% response rate, and 9 of the 10 participants who responded to a single dose of ketamine (the response being measured at 24 hours) continued in the study and received 5 additional infusions on alternate days, over a 2-week period. These patients were only followed up to the final ketamine treatment and had significantly improved at this time. However, given that they were not followed up further, it is not known whether the repeated infusions prevented relapse in this study.

Back in Germany, this time in Munich, another group of researchers led by R. Paul investigated the use of S-ketamine as a single infusion in two patients with treatment-resistant depression, comparing the effects of S-ketamine with racemic ketamine in the same patients.

They found that one patient responded quickly, with the benefit lasting for six days, to both variants of ketamine, whereas one did not respond to either.

Both experienced more side effects from the racemic mixture.[11]

Later, Segmiller et al. in 2013 gave repeated S-ketamine infusions to six patients suffering from treatment-resistant major depression at a rate of 0.25 mg/kg. Each patient received six infusions over three weeks, and they also continued to take their regular medication.

Five of the six improved with this regime although two experienced dissociative side effects.[12]

A field in which pain, anxiety, and depression are highly prevalent is that of palliative care. Here the issues of possible long-term side effects, dependence, and addiction are of secondary importance to rapid and strong symptom relief without major side effects.

Scott Irwin and Alana Iglewicz in the *Journal of Palliative Medicine* in 2010 reported on two patients suffering from terminal illnesses who responded well to the addition of one dose of oral ketamine to their usual medicines.[13]

The first patient they described as a 64-year-old woman suffering from chronic lung disease and respiratory failure. She was oxygen dependent, and her prognosis was poor, with an expected life survival of weeks to a few months at most.

In the prior two months, she had developed symptoms of a full-blown depressive illness with poor sleep, reduced appetite, impaired concentration, excessive guilt, and social withdrawal. She had persistent thoughts about dying but was not actively suicidal. In addition, she experienced panic attacks daily and had become increasingly irritable.

She was given a dose of 27 mg of ketamine in addition to her regular medication. Two hours later, she reported improved mood with reductions in both anxiety symptoms and suicidal thoughts. Subsequently, she became more socially engaged, her appetite improved, her irritability declined, and she was more positive about the future. She described feeling relaxed, more alert, and she described her pain and shortness of breath as improving. She phoned friends and planned social outings. She continued to improve to the extent that her caregiver thanked the team for giving her friend back.

Encouraged by these results, Irwin went on to conduct a more systematic trial in palliative care that I will detail later in this chapter.

Two matters of interest in this report are, first, that Irwin's oral dose was much smaller (a third of that used by Paslakis) and, second, that this single dose appeared to have a lasting impact for both patients.

In 2010 the Charney group led by Sanjay Matthew at the Mount Sinai Hospital in New York released the results of a study in which they initially replicated the original Berman (2000) and Zarate (2006) studies and then tested two compounds that worked on the same brain receptors that ketamine affects.[14] First, they tested riluzole to see if it could prevent relapse after the first successful infusion of ketamine, and they also assessed lamotrigine as a possible enhancer of the immediate mood-elevating effect of ketamine and a reducer of the cognitive and psychomimetic side effects.

They took 26 patients with treatment-resistant depression who were medication-free and gave them 0.5 mg/kg of ketamine intravenously over 40 minutes.

This was a randomised, placebo-controlled, continuation trial, and lamotrigine or a placebo was given just prior to the single treatment with ketamine.

With open-label ketamine, 65% of the patients responded in first 24 hours. The 54% who were still responders after 72 hours were randomised to riluzole or placebo for 32 days, and the time to relapse was measured. This proved to be the same for both treatments, an average of 23 days for both groups.

The treatment was well tolerated, with mild and transient side effects. The pretreatment with lamotrigine had no effect on either the efficacy or the side effects from the ketamine infusion.

The results of the study again confirmed the rapid—and, for some, sustained—effects from a single-dose intravenous infusion of ketamine.

There was no evidence of benefit from the two other medications that affect glutamate receptors.

The response was quite prolonged for some; however, it is possible that this trial recruited patients who had less-severe illnesses than those in the original studies.

In a further study by Ibrahim and Zarate in 2011 at the NIMH, a similar lack of benefit from riluzole given after a ketamine infusion was found. Notably, in their trial, patients who had previously been treated with ECT responded just as well as those who had not.[15]

In contrast to lamotrigine and riluzole, one case study by Kollmar et al. in 2008 found positive results with memantine, another drug acting on the glutamatergic system. In this case study, after failing to maintain an adequate response with two ketamine infusions, the treatment-resistant patient remained well for six months (the final point of follow-up) after commencing 5 mg per day of oral memantine titrated to 15 mg/day over four weeks and remained on this dose in addition to duloxetine, olanzapine, lorazepam, venlafaxine, mirtazapine, and lamotrigine.[16]

The next trial to examine the use of repeated intravenous ketamine infusions was again from Mount Sinai. This team—which included Charney, Matthew, and Rot—took 10 patients from a previous study who had responded to single-dose infusions and gave them 6 doses in total over a period of 12 days, using a similar schedule to giving ECT. The patients were medication-free at the start of the trial. The 9 patients who responded to the first infusion continued to respond after 5 further infusions, with the average time to relapse after the last ketamine dose being 19 days (there was a 6-to-90-day range).[17]

Murrough, Charney, et al. extended this study in 2013 by including the results from the treatment of 14 more patients.

The overall response rate from both studies was 71% and was predicted by a positive two-hour response following the first dose of ketamine.

Three patients reported short-lived dissociative symptoms, and there were other minor side effects including diarrhoea, restlessness, and mild headaches. Brief changes to blood pressure and pulse rates were also noted.[18]

This account established that repeated doses of intravenous ketamine in a group who responded well and quickly to the first dose gave ongoing benefits without untoward side effects.

Nearly all relapsed within three months, again confirming in this treatment-resistant group that ketamine was not a permanent cure.

Overall, the repeated doses were effective and gave longer periods of wellness compared to single doses, and there was no evidence of harm from the ongoing treatment. There were also no signs of tolerance to ketamine's antidepressant effects nor any evidence of dependence or addiction over the time of the study.

In 2010 Diazgranados, Zarate, et al. at the National Institute of Mental Health (NIMH), Bethesda, Maryland, conducted the first trial involving patients with bipolar depression.

This was a randomised, double-blind, single-intravenous-infusion study with a two-week crossover period.

The patients were treatment refractory (resistant), with 55% having previously been given ECT, and they had taken, on average, seven antidepressants to no effect.

Of the 18 patients recruited, 13 completed the study.

Ketamine was added to the mood stabilisers the patients were already taking, namely lithium and sodium valproate. The results showed that a rapid response to ketamine was apparent between 40 minutes after the infusion to day 3 compared with the placebo. The response lasted on average for seven days and the overall response rates for ketamine were 71% versus 6% for the saline placebo.

The treatment was well tolerated, with one episode of hypomania being reported in each group (this episode was limited to the time of infusion in the ketamine group).[19]

Zarate and Diazgranados replicated this study in 2012. At this time, there was a 79% response rate, with decreased suicidal ideation also being evident.[20]

Therapeutic actions of ketamine in bipolar depressed patients

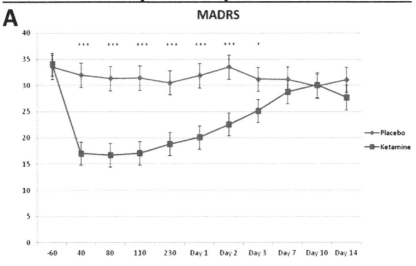

Zarate et al., 2012: Biological Psychiatry

Image courtesy of Ronald Duman

To summarise, there is usually a poor response in bipolar depression to all forms of treatment, particularly with standard antidepressants, and there is also a small risk of triggering a manic episode if they are used alone without the protection of a mood stabiliser.

Therefore, these are important studies establishing that patients with bipolar disorder can indeed benefit from ketamine infusions, and it appears that they responded a little more quickly than unipolar patients.

There was also a clear reduction in suicidal thinking; this occurred rapidly and was not always associated with improved mood. This finding has since been repeated in other studies, including some set in emergency departments.

In 2010 Messer, a physician in behavioural health in Duluth, gave two patients a series of intravenous infusions, with the doses being based on ideal body weight rather than actual body weight, thus avoiding larger doses and increases in side effects that can occur as a consequence. They were both heavy patients weighing 101.8 kg and 159.1 kg respectively.

Over a 12-day period, one patient had six ketamine infusions and the other two, these being given on days 1 and 7 together with four saline infusions.

Both showed a positive rapid response in three to five days. Symptoms returned on day 18 for the patient who had been given two active infusions and day 29 for the patient having six infusions.

The treatment was well tolerated, with a temporary increase in blood pressure and short-lived mild intoxication being noted.

Messer's message was that the amount of ketamine administered needed to be carefully considered as relying on actual rather than ideal body weight could inflate the dosages given with negative consequences.[21]

The following description of one of the patients further illustrates the severity of depressive illnesses for some and the lengths that both patients and their doctors go to in trying to find relief:

> Patient B is a 45-year-old man weighing 101.8 kg (ideal body weight=76.0 kg) with a history of depressive symptoms and treatment since the age of 10. He had been diagnosed with major depressive disorder, resistant type. He also had a history of alcohol abuse. Medical history included diagnoses of hypertension, and he had been treated with nine medications along with ECT. Between 2003 and 2007, this patient received a total of 105 ECT treatments (10 right unilateral treatments, 40 bilateral treatments, 23 modified bilateral treatments, 18 right unilateral/ultrabrief

treatments, and 14 modified bilateral/ultrabrief treatments) and maintenance therapy. Treatment with ECT had produced both short-term and long-term memory loss without full recovery from the depression. In this study, the patient's MMSE score for cognitive function at baseline was in the normal range and no further cognitive testing was pursued. The subject had received implantation of a vagal nerve stimulator, another option for resistant depression, in 2005.

Claudia Zanicotti, in her 2011 thesis written in Dunedin, New Zealand, was one of the first to report the use of intramuscular ketamine for treating depression. Her patient had terminal cancer.

'The results in the case presented in this thesis were positive, with remission of symptoms with single dose and repeated treatment, and maintenance of remission with weekly injections of ketamine 1 mg/kg. This thesis supports the possible use of ketamine as a fast-acting antidepressant in terminal cancer patients with Major Depressive Disorder. In a population with short life expectancy, the existence of a treatment for depressive episodes with rapid onset of action would be essential, and ketamine might be the option of choice.'[22]

She later added in 2012 that, after seven months of weekly doses, her patient had remained well for six months and that she eventually died 'free of depression'. In this situation, there may have been an additive effect from the methadone that her patient was taking as methadone also blocks the NMDA receptor.

It is of interest that she gave ketamine at a higher dose than that later used by Cusin and Chilukiri.

The first report examining the relationship between the different doses of intramuscular injections of ketamine and antidepressant response came from Glue et al. in 2011.[23]

They tested a range of doses (0.5, 0.7, and 1.0 mg/kg) in two patients with treatment-refractory depression. A clear dose response relationship was evident, with the higher doses leading to greater antidepressant response, the average improvement in scores being from 15% (0.5 mg/kg) to 44% (0.7 mg/kg) to 70% (1.0 mg/kg).

Intramuscular ketamine has similar bioavailability (93%) to intravenous ketamine. When given at equal doses to a slow intravenous infusion, intramuscular ketamine had higher peak exposure with the additional benefit of not requiring an infusion pump and being a practical alternative for patients with poor intravenous access.

A second case series from Cusin et al. in 2012 reported the use of repeated doses of intramuscular ketamine for treatment-resistant bipolar II depression.[24]

Two patients were given initial intramuscular injections of ketamine before receiving repeated doses (from 32 to 100 mg every three to four days over several months). This resulted in improved depressive symptoms and, after months of intramuscular administration, the expected side effects of irritability, headaches, nightmares, and dissociation but none of the medical sequelae seen in ketamine abusers (for example, cystitis and liver damage).

They described their first patient as being a 57-year-old woman who had been diagnosed with bipolar II disorder as well as attention deficit disorder. She had experienced recurrent depressive episodes which had not responded to multiple medications and ECT.

She remained on venlafaxine, lamotrigine, and methylphenidate and was started on intravenous ketamine infusions given twice weekly at 0.5 mg/kg over 40 minutes.

After the third infusion, her mood began to improve, but she declined again 19 days after the fifth and final infusion. She was then given oral ketamine at 210 mg per day three times a week for three weeks and then intranasal ketamine at 200 mg/ml three times a week for three weeks; neither of these approaches led to improvement.

She was then given intramuscular ketamine at 32 mg and then at 50 mg and completely remitted after a few days.

She subsequently was given further intramuscular injections when her mood showed signs of decline; on average, this occurred every four days. This schedule was continued for five months, at which time she partially relapsed. Her dose was then increased to 70 mg every four days, and she remained completely asymptomatic for four months. She did experience dissociative symptoms, nightmares, and headaches in the short term following administration.

Apart from the tenacity shown by both patient and doctor, this case demonstrates that ketamine can still be helpful even though one route of administration does not work. Additionally, neither patient had a hypomanic episode during the follow-up despite not being on a mood stabiliser. Neither responded to their first dose of ketamine. There were no reports of the physical side effects (e.g. bladder or cognitive problems described with long-term high-dose ketamine use).

Papolos et al. in 2012 described the use of intranasal ketamine in patients suffering from paediatric bipolar disorder.

He outlined the treatment of 12 youths in a retrospective study of chart records after having treated 40 patients aged 6–19 years with treatment-refractory conditions.

Ketamine substantially reduced symptoms of mania, aggression, and fear of harm. It was well tolerated, and there was a rapid response to doses typically being given every three days.

He would begin with 10 mg of intranasal ketamine, increasing the dose every three to seven days to an effective dose range of 30–120 mg.

All 12 had experienced pretreatment psychotic symptoms, and all had been given prior treatment with mood stabilisers, antipsychotics, and benzodiazepines.

A typical response would be evident within an hour and would last for three to seven days, at which time there would be a dramatic and predictable sequence of symptom return. Side effects were dose dependent. Tolerance to them developed quickly, and they did not last more than an hour after the ketamine was given.

Concurrent medications were gradually withdrawn, and these patients were eventually managed on ketamine alone.

Papolos commented, 'Several findings require further discussion. Ketamine produced rapid improvement of hypomanic and manic hyperactivity, mood lability, hyperarousal, aggressive behaviours and obsessions. Improvement was also seen in ratings of anxiety, sleep, inattention, racing thoughts and carbohydrate craving. In most cases we observed a complete abolishment of manic/hypomanic and depressive symptoms. Ketamine administration also led to remission of symptoms associated with the core features of the FOH phenotype, including fear of harm, sleep-onset and sleep-offset disturbances, parasomnias, and the thermoregulatory symptoms associated with this syndrome.'[25]

A more formal prospective study is under way to further clarify these findings. If replicated, they will prove to be of utmost importance, particularly in demonstrating that ketamine can be safely used for extended periods in this age group. Also significant is that it can be used alone as a treatment, reducing the long-term side effects that can occur with other medications. Given that hypomanic and manic symptoms were not made worse by its use but in fact improved with ketamine, treatment of elevated mood states could be extended to adult populations with bipolar disorder. Could it be that ketamine is a mood stabiliser rather than an antidepressant?

Szymkowicz and colleagues in 2012 described the courses of 3 patients given intravenous ketamine over a 12-month period. All had long histories of treatment resistance, were on medication, and were due for ECT.

They were treated initially as inpatients, then were followed up as outpatients once they responded. The plan was to give six treatments, initially every second day, then further doses as necessary when there were signs of relapse.

All three made patchy progress after the initial successful course of treatment, but ketamine did prove to be helpful. One patient took four infusions to respond, and another needed seven infusions.

They reported that the first patient had a long history of major depression with co-morbid panic disorder and had made multiple suicide attempts over the past 20 years. Through the years, she had failed to respond to trials of 20 different antidepressants, but fortunately, she did obtain relief from ECT, having 35 treatments over 3 separate courses. However, the ECT had been associated with significant cognitive impairment, which had contributed to her losing work. At the time of her current admission, which was triggered by her attempt to hang herself, she was taking fluoxetine (an antidepressant), lamotrigine (a mood stabiliser), quetiapine (an antipsychotic), and lorazepam (an anti-anxiety agent).

She was commenced on 27 mg of intravenous ketamine given over 40 minutes and, 4 hours later, had experienced complete relief of her depressive symptoms. Her mood remained stable, and after a further infusion four days later, she was discharged. Eight days later, she described mild depressive symptoms and was given a further infusion, again improving. She then had further treatments at lengthening intervals, eventually receiving doses seven weeks apart. After eight months, a series of life events, including a failed relationship, triggered a relapse, and she received three treatments of ketamine in close order, which again showed clear benefit. After 12 months, she was taking substantially lower doses of fluoxetine and quetiapine and was only using the lorazepam when required. Over the 12-month period, she had received 16 infusions of ketamine without troublesome side effects; in particular, she showed no signs of cognitive impairment.

This treatment approach of waiting for signs of relapse and then treating quickly does avoid unnecessary use of ketamine, but it does require accurate self-monitoring from patients and the ready availability of therapy.

In 2012 McNulty[27] outlined his work with a patient in palliative care. This single-case report is notable for its initial use of subcutaneous ketamine (later to be assessed by Colleen Loo and her group in Australia, then used by Graham Barrett at the Aura Medical Centres), followed by daily oral ketamine.

He outlined his management of a 44-year-old hospice patient with a terminal illness who was experiencing severe chronic pain together with anxiety and depressive symptoms, none of which had been relieved by standard treatments. He was given a single subcutaneous 0.5 mg dose of ketamine, which provided him with immediate and substantial relief for 80 hours. He was then given oral ketamine daily, this being flavoured to mask the bitterness of the ketamine, and continued to benefit without problematical side effects.

Next, in 2012 in Canada came a case report from Blier et al.,[28] who described the management of a 44-year-old patient with treatment-resistant depression who received more than 40 ketamine infusions over several months. Although her depression initially abated and there were no observed cognitive deficits, ketamine was not as efficacious on repeated dosing, possibly indicating a diminishing response to ketamine.

From India in 2013, Harihar Chilukuri et al.[29] described in a follow-up case series of two patients with depression, a rapid antidepressant response to intramuscular ketamine. In this situation, ECT was being considered, but because the students had exams pending, the decision was made to try the ketamine first. The effect of the first injection lasted for a week, and both students responded well to further injections.

Their first patient—a single, male 23-year-old medical student— had a five-year history of obsessive-compulsive disorder with obscene thoughts, excessive guilt, and depressive episodes.

After admitting to thoughts of suicide, he had been commenced on a combination of the antidepressants fluoxetine and bupropion but subsequently had attempted to cut his throat and was sent for psychiatric review.

At the time of assessment, he was actively suicidal, and a course of ECT was discussed. However, as he had exams pending and there were concerns about ECT's effects on memory, he agreed to a trial of ketamine and was given 0.5 mg intramuscularly. He had no significant side effects and, two hours later, reported a marked improvement in mood and cessation of his suicidal thoughts. Three days later, he was given a further dose of ketamine, and he again described improvement. He continued to take his antidepressant medication and, a month later, had maintained his remission and took his final exams, 'doing well to his satisfaction'.

In 2014 Harihar and his colleagues compared three regimes of ketamine, one of 0.5 mg/kg intravenously, the second using the same dose intramuscularly, and the third using a half-strength (0.25 mg/kg) intramuscular dose. There were nine patients in each group, and patients were randomised. This was an open-label design, and patients remained on their usual medications. On average, there was a 60% reduction in depression scores in all three groups, this being evident two hours after the injections, and the improvement persisted for three days.[30]

In 2013 Irwin, who had detailed the effects of adding a low dose of oral ketamine to the regular medications of two palliative-care patients in 2010, presented a study of 14 patients in palliative care treated with oral ketamine for 28 days.[31] Of the 14 patients who started, 8 completed the study, 2 withdrew for non-trial-related reasons, and 4 were non-responders.

Daily oral ketamine at a dose of 0.5 mg/kg was added to the patients' current medication. Rare and mild side effects, including diarrhoea, sleep disturbance, and restlessness were described. The eight completers all had significant improvements in both anxiety and depressive symptoms.

The response was evident by day 3 for anxiety and by day 14 for depression. This delayed antidepressant effect contrasted with their previous experience of positive responses from a single dose. The effect on anxiety symptoms was also notable, and more recently, there have been trials in patients with obsessive-compulsive disorder and post-traumatic stress disorder that had positive results.

A further extension of this work by Iglewicz and Irwin will be published later in 2015.[32] Curiously, in this report, patients responded quickly to the introduction of ketamine.

They described a retrospective chart study of 31 hospice patients who had been given oral ketamine, examining degrees of improvement, time to improvement, and side effects.

They noted that, of those responding to ketamine, 93% did so in the first three days and the majority of patients had experienced either no side effects or only mild side effects that did not impair function.

In 2013 Messer described the use of maintenance ketamine in a single-case report.[33] He used intravenous ketamine and followed the patient for close to two years, one of the longest follow-up periods yet described.

> The first Ketamine treatment led to a dramatic remission of depressive symptoms: the Beck Depression Inventory (BDI) score decreased from 22 to 6. Three additional infusions administered every other day over 5 days produced remission lasting 17 days after the last dose in this series.
>
> Three further series of six ketamine infusions given every other day except weekends were given over the next 16 weeks. Each infusion sequence produced remission lasting 16, 28, and 16 days, respectively, followed by a relapse. After three remission/relapse cycles and before relapse could occur after the fourth infusion series, a maintenance ketamine regimen was established on August 27, 2008 using 0.5 mg/kg IBW [ideal body weight] at a 3-week inter-dose interval. The authors' estimation for the maintenance-dosing interval was based on the average time frame between remission and relapse for this patient. Relapse to depression was prevented by treating prior to the onset of a relapse.
>
> With maintenance infusions the patient has been in remission for more than 15 months. No concurrent pharmacotherapeutic agents have been administered or

required during this time period, no adverse events have emerged, and there has been no cognitive impairment as is typical with ECT and polypharmacy.

Messer's approach to maintenance ketamine is similar to that employed with patients who respond to ECT but then relapse within a predictable period. In this situation, ECT is given prophylactically to try to prevent the drop in mood.

In recent years, online forums have provided increasing amounts of information about both the recreational and the medical use of ketamine. The quality of the content is amazingly varied, but it is always interesting to read.

Foreigner posted on Bluelight's ketamine forum in 2013:[34]

THE REGIMEN.

The regimen lasted 7 days and was performed with intramuscular injection (IM). If you can't set this up to be IM then it's going to be difficult to precisely regulate your intake and in my opinion there would be no point in attempting this, but others may disagree and I have spoken with those who have used the snorting ROA [route of administration] with success.

The goal, based on research and anecdotal reports of others who have personally done this regimen, was to maintain the alteration of consciousness similar to having drunk one beer. You bring yourself to the threshold of onset with each dose, without actually triggering the psychedelic experience. If you do this, you will benefit from the nootropic effect [can improve memory, motivation, and attention and is literally mind bending]. If you take the psychedelic dose, you will achieve the opposite and suffer ketamine abuse side effects. Heed this warning: do not succumb to the desire to do higher doses or to dose more often. It will compromise your therapy.

The goal is to maintain threshold ketamine levels in your brain so that the NMDA receptors remain saturated but not over-stimulated. You will know that saturation is being achieved because eventually hourly doses won't feel like they are doing much. Even the light buzz with each dose is no longer all that present. In my case, day 3 was when this happened. At this point you can begin spacing out the doses to every two hours, followed by every three hours, and then finally every four hours. One individual I connected with said they took 10 mg every hour basically running around. I had to keep a close eye on the clock and find the nearest washroom to take a dose. This made things completely chaotic (not to mention legally risky) and if I had my time back I wouldn't have done it, but c'est la vie, a.k.a shit happens. As an aside: major respect to people who have addictions that require them to dose in potentially risky locations!

In 2014 Foreigner posted an update saying that he had experienced a return of depressive symptoms following a major move and had taken a single 10 mg dose of ketamine intramuscularly, finding immediate relief. He now considers that his depressive episodes are not a result of underlying unresolved emotional issues but that he has an ongoing brain dysfunction that cannot be permanently fixed. He sees ketamine as not being a cure for his condition as he had originally hoped, but he remains grateful for finding something that works and continues to be effective for him. His main wish is that doctors in Canada would agree to prescribe ketamine so that he does not have to continue to obtain it illegally.

Foreigner's use of a continuous dosing schedule through his waking hours hearkens back to the original work by Correll and Futter with their five-day infusions and certainly is an approach that merits further study.

In 2013 Murrough et al. published a single-dose trial of intravenous ketamine compared with intravenous midazolam in 72 medication-free patients with treatment-resistant depression.[35] This work was conducted in two centres and attempted to deal with one of the biggest problems with the earlier double-blind trials. Because of ketamine's effects on the brain, it is quite possible that patients and researchers could guess who had been given the ketamine rather than placebo, and this may have influenced their expectations of benefit.

Midazolam, which is used as a short-acting anaesthetic, shares some effects with ketamine, and the group hoped that this would be a more valid placebo.

The response 24 hours after the ketamine infusion was positive for 64% of those who were given ketamine compared to 28% for those who received midazolam.

Of the original 47 who received ketamine, 21 were still responders at 7 days compared to 4 of the 25 who were given midazolam.

FIGURE 2. Response Rates Over Time in Patients With Treatment-Resistant Major Depression Given a Single In- fusion of Ketamine or Midazolam[a]

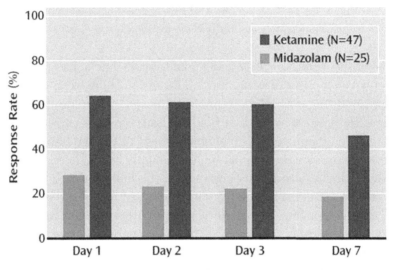

[a] Modified intention-to-treat group. Response at each time point was defined as a decrease from baseline of at least 50% in score on the Montgomery-Åsberg Depression Rating Scale.

Am J Psychiatry. 2013 Oct 1;170(10):1134-42.Antidepressant efficacy of ketamine in treatment-resistant major depression: a two-site randomized controlled trial. Murrough JW et al

On the positive side, this was a comparatively large study conducted in two sites using a psychoactive placebo not known to be an antidepressant showing a clear result in favour of ketamine. On the negative side, patients still may have been able to pick the difference; it would be very difficult to find a drug that could mimic all of ketamine's effects.

In 2013 Rasmussen and Lineberry from the Mayo Clinic, Rochester, reported on their use of ketamine in ten patients with treatment-resistant depression.[36] They gave serial intravenous ketamine infusions given twice weekly with a minimum of four treatments. There was a four-week follow-up.

To reduce side effects and the need for intensive anaesthetic monitoring, they gave the ketamine at a lower dose than usual (0.3 mg/kg) over a longer time of 100 minutes.

There was an 80% response rate and a 50% remission rate, and tolerability was good, with mild side effects limited to the infusion period.

Only one patient remitted after the first dose; this again contradicted the prevailing idea that, for intravenous ketamine, early strong responses predicted long-term outcomes. In this study, multiple infusions were more effective than single doses. They stated that, by giving a lower dose for longer, they were able to significantly reduce the cost and complexity of treatment as, at their institution, a higher dose required full anaesthetic monitoring. They also considered that the slower infusion rate would give fewer side effects.

They further speculated that daily infusions would be possible with this lower-dose strategy. They argued that the main reason ECT is not usually given daily is the concern about a build-up of cognitive side effects, which would make it difficult to judge improvement, but with ketamine, this has not been an issue in their experience.

It is interesting that the usual spacing of serial ketamine treatments has followed the ECT model of alternate-day dosing. Perhaps this is not the most effective approach?

In 2013 Diogo Lara and colleagues from the Pontifícia Universidade Católica do Rio Grande do Sul, Porto Alegre, Brazil, and the Hospital Espírita de Marília, Marília, Brazil, reported on the use of sublingual ketamine for treatment-resistant patients.[37]

This was an open-label trial, and they gave 26 patients with either unipolar or bipolar conditions very low doses of ketamine every 2–7 days. Both patients and their relatives reported rapid and sustained effects, with a 77% response rate and very few side effects.

The first dose was 10 mg and was held under the tongue for three to four minutes; this compares with the usual starting dose for an intravenous infusion of 35 mg.

Given these outstanding results, it is very important that this study, particularly the response to ultra-low doses, be replicated and Lara is currently organising an open-label inpatient trial. It was this study that persuaded me to try this approach with my patients; two of them have improved at these very low starting doses, but the majority has needed, on average, 50 mg of ketamine sublingually to establish a good response. More information about Lara's study is available in chapter 7, 'The Ketamine Doctors'.

Moving from the ultra-low doses of ketamine to the other extreme, we have a report from Delisa Guadarrama, MD, which was presented at the APA annual meeting in 2013, on the use of intravenous ketamine at the rate of 2 mg/kg body weight to treat severe postpartum depression and other depressive disorders. She explained that the infusions were given in a pain clinic that was accustomed to using these doses. Interestingly, the response to a single treatment persisted for three weeks or more in contrast to the one-week duration of effect commonly found with the 0.5 mg/kg dose, and the level of side effects was similar.[38]

Again exploring different routes of administration in 2014, Lapidus et al. from the Mount Sinai group used intranasal ketamine at a dose of 50 mg compared to a saline placebo in a randomised, double-blind, crossover trial.[39]

At 24 hours post treatment, 44% of the ketamine group had responded as opposed to 6% in the placebo group. Side effects were mild and short term.

Although the reported benefit was lower than most others using a single treatment, the study showed that the intranasal route was a practical option at least for short-term treatment.

Also in 2014, Jaskaran Singh, who works at Janssen Pharmaceuticals, reported in a poster session that, in a study of 67 patients given intravenous ketamine for treatment-resistant depression, there was a good overall response better than placebo. Interestingly, there was no significant difference in response between those given infusions twice a week and those given them three times a week over a four-week period.[40]

The first report from a United Kingdom study of ketamine treatment for depression came from Diamond, McShane, et al. from Oxford. In 2014 they described a trial of intravenous ketamine in 28 patients with treatment-resistant unipolar and bipolar depressive conditions.[41]

They were interested in assessing whether the memory problems seen in some patients following ECT would be a problem after repeated treatment with ketamine.

Their patients were given 3–6 infusions of 0.5 mg/kg ketamine in 40 minutes over a 3-week period, and they noted that only 3 of 8 responders had done so before their second infusion. Their patients had continued to take their pretreatment medication. After 3 weeks, 29% had responded, 14% had remitted, and 15% took 2 months or more to relapse. They added that they had now treated 45 patients (400 infusions) and that 20% of those treated had sufficient benefits to warrant having ongoing infusions. Over 2 years of ongoing treatment, there had been no indications of dependence or addiction. Nor was there evidence of bladder inflammation or memory loss, issues that are experienced by long-term, high-dose ketamine addicts.

Dr McShane says:

> We've seen remarkable changes in people who've had severe depression for many years that no other treatment has touched. It's very moving to witness. Patients often comment that that the flow of their thinking seems suddenly freer. For some, even a brief experience of response helps them to realise that they can get better and this gives hope.
>
> In summary, this case series suggests that ketamine infusions in treatment resistant depression can be given safely to patients who remain on antidepressants, but that they can occasionally cause marked acute anxiety, vomiting and vasovagal episodes. Potential problems regarding cognitive function were not realised. The ECT clinic appeared to offer an appropriate level of acute monitoring and supervision for initial infusions. Ketamine has complex effects on suicidality, and may cause mood instability, which requires careful monitoring. Our experience raises the possibilities that its dramatic and useful antidepressant effect may require at least two infusions to become apparent and last longer if taken with other antidepressants, but clearly more work is needed to confirm this.

Meanwhile, people continued to share information through the World Wide Web. Cathy, a contributor to Medchat.com, an online forum, said in 2014:[42]

> I have been taking 1.6 mg/kg of ketamine orally once every three to five days for the past three months. The effects have been dramatic. Yes, there is a period for about 1–2 hours after taking it that you feel weird, not worried, but weird. That effect can vary each time, and changes.
>
> I currently take between 1.6 and 2 mg/kg ketamine as an oral/sublingual syrup once every three to five days. It is doing wonders for my anxiety and generally working well for the depression. Note that I am taking to medication orally/sublingually, which is different from how most patients in the U.S. take it. The anxiety effect tends to last at least three days, the antidepressant effect at some points in my menstrual cycle only last 2 days. So I am learning what depression without anxiety feels like, and also to identify what are early warning signs that the drug is wearing off. If you have control over timing of treatments you want to space them out as far as possible while still preventing the depression from recurring, and taking as low a dose as possible . . .
>
> Best wishes to you. I hope you find some help either with ketamine, with physical or cognitive/behavioural therapy, or with something like rTMS, or DCTCS [new brain stimulation treatments]. There are new pharmaceuticals in development based on ketamine. Hang in there, eventually something will work.

In 2014 P. Clark, who works in a private practice in Carolina, detailed in a case report the use of intranasal ketamine at a dose of 50 mg twice weekly in a treatment-resistant patient.[43]

Her patient was a 44-year-old woman with a ten-year history of recurrent major depression and migraine and had required several hospitalisations. In the past, she had not responded well to antidepressant medication but had obtained partial relief from courses of ECT. Despite taking a combination of antidepressants and antipsychotics for her current episode, she did not improve and began to voice suicidal thoughts. She declined a further trial of ECT, so Dr Clark attempted to enrol her in a ketamine research trial. However, as the need was becoming urgent, she referred her to a neurologist who treated refractory migraine using intranasal ketamine, the hope being that ketamine would help both conditions. Her patient was given intranasal ketamine at a dose of 50 mg twice weekly for four months.

She showed partial improvement after three days and then progressed to full remission over the next two weeks. Her mood remained stable over a four-month period, and she was able to return to work. Side effects were mild and well tolerated, with brief euphoria described after the first few treatments.

From Australia in 2014, Gálvez, Loo, et al. described in a case report the use of subcutaneous [SC] ketamine for treating depression.[44] The subcutaneous route is thought to give similar blood levels to intravenous ketamine, and the dose is easier to administer.

Their patient was a 62-year-old woman with recurrent unipolar major depressive disorder. In her current episode, after failing to respond to antidepressant medication nortriptyline, she declined ECT and was given ketamine as part of a research trial.

'She was given treatments of ketamine .1 mg/kg, midazolam .01 mg/kg (as active placebo), and ketamine .2 mg/kg (weight: 72 kg), given in that order, administered via abdominal SC injection, with treatment sessions separated by 3 weeks and 1 week, respectively. Her response to .1 mg/kg lasted 2 weeks. After treatment with .2 mg/kg ketamine, she remained in remission without residual symptoms for 5 months, while continuing on a regimen of nortriptyline.'

They noted that her ketamine doses were well tolerated, with reported side effects being mild light-headedness and blurred vision starting at 5 minutes after injection and resolving by 40–60 minutes.

She relapsed after 5 months and, on this occasion, received 12 treatments of SC ketamine at 0.2 mg/kg. She improved after 3 ketamine treatments but did not attain a lasting response until 12 treatments were given. Ketamine was again well tolerated. After her last treatment session, the patient remained in remission for more than ten weeks and was being actively followed up.

They concluded that the advantages of the subcutaneous route included simplicity and less pain than that experienced with intravenous and intramuscular injections and better bioavailability of ketamine compared to the oral route.

In 2014 Nguyen et al reported the results of a retrospective chart review of 18 patients who had been treated with ketamine solution placed on the top of their tongues ["transmucosal administration"]. [45]

They had been diagnosed with treatment-resistant depression and treated by one of the co-authors Scott Pollard at the Chestnut Ridge Day Hospital facility in Morgantown, USA.

The mean age of the patients was 48. They were given ketamine 0.5 – 1 mg/kg bodyweight, this being added to their usual medications, which included antidepressants and stimulants.

The dose was initially administered every 14 days and then varied according to progress. Overall they described a response rate of 76%.

Significantly these were "dirty" patients, having multiple co-morbidities, unlike those who are usually selected for clinical trials. There were transient symptoms of headaches and dizziness noted, but no ongoing adverse effects.

In 2015 Hu et al from the University of Macau published the results of a trial of combining a single dose of intravenous ketamine with a newly initiated antidepressant, escitalopram. [46]

They randomised 30 patients with "severe" depression to receive a single dose of either intravenous ketamine at 0.5mg/kg bodyweight or saline, with both groups then being given escitalopram 10mg daily for 28 days.

The ketamine group showed a 92% response rate and a 57% remission rate, whereas the saline group had a 57% response rate and a 14% remission rate.

The ketamine group also responded and remitted more quickly with improved rating scores being evident 2 hours post-infusion and at 2 weeks. Measures of suicidal ideation were significantly improved in the ketamine group both at 2 hours and 72 hours post-infusion.

There were no ongoing adverse effects noted in either group.

Zhang et al replicated this study in 2018 with 82 patients being randomised and a response rate of 90% and a remission rate of 71% being reported in the ketamine group. These results were significantly better from 2 hours post-infusion onward compared to the control group. [47] Their patients were described as having "depression" and it is probable that neither this study nor the preceding Hu study included treatment-resistant patients. This could well have contributed to the comparatively high success rates.

Y Domani et al from Tel Aviv reported in 2016 on a comparison of oral ketamine versus placebo in a double-blind, randomised, controlled trial for patients with treatment-resistant depression.[48] Their 22 patients took doses daily. Those taking ketamine showed a rapid response and their improvement measured at 21 days was significantly better than placebo. They described ketamine as being well tolerated.

I have not yet been able to access details of the trial nor the doses used.

Jasfarinia and colleagues from Tehran published a paper in 2016 comparing the efficacy of oral ketamine and diclofenac [an anti-inflammatory medication] monotherapy in depressed patients who were also experiencing chronic pain.[49]

This was a double-blind, randomised, controlled trial that was conducted over 6 weeks and enrolled 40 patients.

They were given either 150mg of diclofenac or 150mg of ketamine orally daily for 6 weeks.

Those in the ketamine group showed significantly improved depression scores compared to the diclofenac group. Interestingly there was a greater effect noted in the ketamine group at 6 weeks compared to the same patients at 3 weeks, reinforcing the need for longer durations of therapy for some. Also, there was no significant difference in pain reduction between the two medications.

Ketamine was well tolerated.

Lenze et al at the Washington University School of Medicine St. Louis extended the work of Corell and Futter published in 2006 with the following pilot study.[50] They compared 10 patients with TRD who were randomised with one group given a continuous infusion of ketamine over 96 hours and a second group of 10 being given one dose of ketamine intravenously over the final 40 minutes of a 96-hour saline infusion.

Both groups were given oral clonidine to see if this would reduce both the elevations of pulse rate and blood pressure often seen with intravenous ketamine therapy and also the psychotomimetic effects.

Patients were followed for 8 weeks with rapid and sustained improvement in mood being noted in both groups and there were no significant adverse effects reported.

At 24 hours post-infusion 7out of 10 patients in both groups had responded.

There was a numerical advantage apparent with the continuous infusion patients at both 2 weeks and 8 weeks, but this did not reach statistical significance – the small numbers in each group meant the study was not adequately powered to detect a difference.

There was slight lowering of BP attributable to the clonidine, but no rebound when this was ceased.

Psychotomimetic effects were mild and transient in both groups and did not correlate with ketamine concentrations. However, in the 96-hour infusion group higher ketamine concentrations did correlate with clinical improvement. Importantly there were no liver enzyme elevations, which have occasionally been noted with repeated long-term ketamine infusions for patients with pain conditions.

This study demonstrates both the feasibility and the safety of this approach and trials with both greater numbers and the inclusion of a group not taking clonidine are clearly warranted. Interestingly a prolonged infusion-like approach involving people self-administering ketamine hourly for 3-4 days then ceasing and observing progress is a strategy sometimes discussed in online patient forums.

On a larger scale altogether we have this 2017 study by Cohen et al in the USA on adverse events from the FDA reporting system which showed that for 40,000 patients given ketamine for pain there was a 50% reduction in depressive symptoms reported compared to those who used other pain medicines.[51]

Notably from this study, diclofenac and minocycline also showed antidepressant effects, albeit to a lesser degree than the ketamine. The data indicated increased renal and liver function effects in the ketamine group emphasising the need for caution in those with renal and hepatic impairment. Reduced opioid side effects were also evident in those taking both opiates and ketamine in combination for pain conditions.

The majority of the early ketamine trials used fixed dose regimes. In actual clinical practice and with most medicines dosing is flexible reflecting both differences in severity of illness and individual differences in absorption, metabolism and overall responsiveness.

To explore the effects of differential dosing the following 2017 study from Australia authored by George, Loo et al entitled "A Pilot Randomised Controlled Trial of Titrated Subcutaneous Ketamine In Older Patients With Treatment-Resistant Depression." appeared in the American Journal of Geriatric Psychiatry in November 2017. [52]

This was a double-blind, randomised, controlled study of 16 patients aged 60 and over suffering from treatment-resistant depression.

They were given increasing doses of subcutaneous ketamine [0.1,0.2,0.3,0.4,0.5 mg/kg bodyweight] weekly over 5 weeks with an active placebo [midazolam] being randomly inserted for one dose.

After the controlled phase 12 further treatments in an open-label phase were given both for non-remitters and those who had relapsed.

After the RCT phase there was a 43% remission rate [7 of 14 completers] and 5 of the 7 remitted at doses below 0.5mg/kg.

Overall, there was 68.8% response rate and ketamine was well tolerated without problematic side effects. Multiple doses were associated with increasing remission rates and longer intervals to relapse.

They concluded that these response and remission rates were similar to those reported in younger populations.

In a similar vein Carolina Da Frota, in her review of ketamine use in the elderly in 2017, described its beneficial effect on two patients given ongoing infusions over time. [53] Clearly age is no barrier to success -the oldest patient I've been involved with who has found ketamine effective is now 90.

Colleen Loo and associates are currently conducting a 200 patient, randomised, controlled trial in seven centres in Australia and New Zealand. This large-scale study has been publicly funded and includes both a double-blind phase where subcutaneous ketamine is given twice weekly for 4 weeks to patients with treatment-resistant depression and also a continuation phase.

Another retrospective study published in 2017 came from Al Shirawi et al in the Journal of Clinical Psychopharmacology.[54] They examined the records of 22 patients with treatment-resistant depression who had failed at least 3 adequate antidepressant trials and one adequate trial of repetitive transcranial magnetic stimulation.

They received open-label treatment with oral ketamine commencing with at a dose of 50 mg taken every 3 days with this then being titrated up by 25 mg every 3 days, according to response and tolerability. The upper dose limit was 300mg.

Over the course of treatment 18% of the patients showed greater than 50% reduction in the Beck Depression Inventory II scores, 14% reported partial improvement in mood symptoms, while 45% had no response to ketamine and 23% showed a mild worsening in their depressive symptoms.

Ketamine was well tolerated, but with only 30% of patients reporting some benefit these results are less impressive than most other studies to date. Perhaps the upper dose limit of 300mg every 3 days was insufficient for these patients. There are also indications from the inclusion criteria that this was a more severely ill group than those in most other studies which only require two failed treatments before patients qualify to try ketamine. If we were to treat this group with another standard antidepressant we would anticipate around a 10% response rate as evidenced by the Star D trial.

The next exploration by Cusin et al in 2017 involved firstly giving 14 patients with treatment-resistant depression intravenous ketamine at the standard dose of 0.5mg/kg bodyweight for 3 treatments and then increasing the dose to 0.75mg/kg for a further 3 treatments. The duration of the ketamine trial was 3 weeks and the ketamine was added to current antidepressant therapy.[55]

After the first 3 doses one of the 14 had responded, after the 6th dose five had responded and two remitted. In the 3 month follow up one sustained the response while the others relapsed within 2 weeks. The treatment was well tolerated.

These patients were more typical of those seen normal clinical practice in that they had high comorbidities and had failed many treatments [42% had failed previous courses of ECT].

This study indicated that repeated doses of ketamine are needed for many to establish the likelihood of response, that increasing the dose is often necessary and that ongoing ketamine therapy is required to maintain improvement for the more complex patients.

Continuing the theme of differential dosing we have a study by Papakostas and Fava from the MGH Clinical Trials Network and Institute published in 2017.[56]

They recruited 99 patients with treatment-resistant depression who were randomly assigned to groups receiving either single doses of 0.1,0.2,0.5 and 1.0 mg /kg bodyweight of intravenous ketamine or the active placebo midazolam. Both groups were assessed for improvement at 24 hours post-infusion and then at 3 days.

Combining the different ketamine dose scores revealed a statistically significant improvement over the active placebo with the benefit being strongest at 24 hours. When examined separately the higher doses had both stronger beneficial effects and more side effects.

Back in Tehran Arabzadeh, Jasfarinia et al have explored whether oral ketamine added to sertraline accelerated treatment response in patients suffering from major depression. This was a double-blind, controlled trial published in February 2018 in the journal of Affective Disorders.[57]

There had previously been a number of case reports suggesting that oral ketamine started simultaneously with conventional antidepressants could speed up recovery.

The researchers enrolled 81 patients with moderate to severe depression [not treatment-resistant] and looked for effects at 2, 4 and 6 weeks after initiation. Patients built up to 150mg daily of sertraline and were given either 50mg a day of ketamine or a placebo for 6 weeks.

At all three time points there was a significant improvement noted in the ketamine versus the placebo group. Early improvement [at 2 weeks] in the sertraline plus ketamine group was 85.4% compared to 42.5% in the sertraline plus placebo group. At six weeks 85.4% were responders to ketamine and sertraline group as opposed to 57.5% in the placebo plus sertraline group. There were neither any significant difference in side effects noted nor any indication of ketamine misuse.

An interesting further investigation would involve adding ketamine only, sertraline only and placebo only groups and/or using a once only larger oral dose of ketamine to compare with the Hu and Zhang studies.

Papolos, who released a paper in 2012 concerning his management of paediatric bipolar disorder, has recently updated progress in this group with a retrospective chart review. [58]

He reported that intranasal ketamine, at a mean dose of 165mg every 3-4 days, had been taken by 45 treatment-resistant patients for periods ranging from 3 months to 6.5 years.

Benefits have been sustained with marked reduction in CGI scores.

The treatment was tolerable with time-limited adverse effects, the intensity of which diminished over time without loss of benefit.

Reported side effects included sensory problems, urination problems, torso acne, dizziness and "wobbly" gait.

This study, taken in conjunction with Cullen's work [described next] which studied administering intravenous ketamine to adolescents, gives greater confidence that ketamine therapy can be both safe and effective in this age group. In particular Papolos has shown that ketamine can be safely used over the longer term which is in accord with reports from many treating adult patients including Angelo de Gioannis, Steve Levine, Glen Brooks, Steve Mandel Varun Jaitly and Lucinda Grande [see Ketamine doctors, Chapter 7] and from my own experience since 2014 of treating 35 patients.

Cullen et al reported in 2018 that they had given 13 adolescents [aged 12-18 years] with treatment-resistant depression 6 intravenous infusions of ketamine over 2 weeks.[59] Those with bipolar diagnoses were excluded in contrast to the Papolos report.

The 5 patients who were given doses of ketamine based on ideal bodyweight did not respond whereas 5 of the 8 whose doses were based on actual bodyweight did. The treatment was well tolerated.

By comparison Papolos reported effective doses as varying widely between 20-360mg taken intranasally every 3-4 days.

Cullen commented that in general children require higher doses of ketamine to develop dissociative symptoms, suggesting they may require higher doses generally and also that it is likely that early onset depression is more severe and less responsive to therapy than mature onset conditions.

Of the recently published studies one of the more significant is that from Angelo De Gioannis and colleagues from Brisbane, Australia. [60] Their work appeared in The Journal Of Psychopharmacology and was published online in November 2017. It was titled "Impact of oral ketamine augmentation on hospital admissions in treatment-resistant depression and PTSD: A retrospective study," and in the paper they compared hospitalisation rates and hospital bed days for a group of 37 patients who were being treated with oral ketamine in December 2015. They examined the data for equivalent periods before and after initiating ketamine therapy and also looked for adverse medical events and changes in ketamine dosage over time.

They found that hospital bed days were reduced by 70% in these patients, some of whom took ketamine for up to 3 years. In addition, hospital admissions were reduced by 65%.

Importantly there were no serious adverse effects experienced either in the short or longer term. Notably there was no evidence of tolerance building over time with doses of ketamine, if anything, decreasing during the maintenance phase.

Angelo and his colleagues have now treated more than 800 patients with oral ketamine over the past 6 years in their outpatient setting with efficacy rates equivalent to those seen with the intravenous route and at significantly lower cost. These findings are particularly relevant for governments and insurers trying to contain the spiralling costs of hospital care.

Further information on Angelo's work can be found in Chapter 7 – "The Ketamine Doctors."

There have been two recent meta-analyses exploring the use of ketamine in combination with electroconvulsive therapy for depression. One suggested a positive effect, the other concluded that adding ketamine made no difference.

This recent study by Gamble et al from Canada will have doubting clinicians thinking again.[61]

They had planned to recruit 72 patients for their study comparing ECT with ketamine anaesthesia to ECT with another standard anaesthetic, propofol. Demographic and clinical data did not vary between the 2 groups. After 12 patients in each group were treated the trial was halted on the advice of the ethics committee.

Twelve patients were given ketamine at a dose of 0.75mg/kg bodyweight along with adjunctive remifentanil [an opiate sedative] and succinylcholine [a muscle relaxant] – both commonly used for ECT anaesthesia. The second group of twelve was given propofol along with the same doses of adjunctive medications. There was no need for extra anaesthesia recorded. The mean number of treatments leading to response was 2 in the ketamine group compared to 4 in the propofol group. All 12 in the ketamine group remitted compared to 7 in the propofol group. The mean number of treatments leading to remission was 3 for the ketamine group and 7 for the propofol group. Side effects were similar in both groups and the duration of seizures in both groups exceeded 15 seconds, indicating adequate brain stimulation. Over the 30 days post treatment one patient in each of the groups relapsed.

The study was terminated early on ethical grounds, given the clear superiority of the ketamine therapy. The authors commented that previous studies had often used different combinations of anaesthetic agents, which may have modified the action of ketamine and/or the quality and duration of the convulsions. In one prior negative study using ketamine as the main anaesthetic the dose of ketamine used was significantly higher which may also have affected the outcome.

Given the mixed results reported to date it is very important that this study be replicated. Significantly there is an ongoing study by Anand in Cleveland Ohio, which is directly comparing treatment with ketamine alone versus ECT over 3 weeks. This study follows that by Ghasemi et al in 2013 showing superiority over 3 treatments for ketamine infusions versus ECT in an 18 patient study.[62]

Albott et al explored the issue of comorbidity in their 2018 paper published in Clinical Psychiatry.[63] They examined the use of ketamine in 15 patients diagnosed with both treatment-resistant depression [TRD] and posttraumatic stress disorder [PTSD]. They were given 6 intravenous infusions of 0.5mg/kg bodyweight ketamine over 12 days with an 8-week follow up phase after the final infusion during which weekly assessments were made. For PTSD symptoms 12 patients remitted with a median relapse time of 41 days and for the TRD symptoms 14 responded with a median time of 20 days to relapse.

Transient dissociation during the infusion occurred, however there was no worsening of PTSD symptoms. Dissociation is a frequent symptom of PTSD so there had been concern about this given ketamine's propensity to induce dissociative symptoms.

Most patients seen in clinical practice have a number of physical and psychological comorbidities making therapy more complex and worsening outcomes. By contrast clinical trials often exclude those with comorbid conditions which can result in higher rates of response and remission being achieved. With this in mind it is good to see that both disorders responded in this small open label trial.

Davis et al reported on the results of ketamine therapy for 54 patients treated at Yale between 2014 and 2017 – they were not part of a clinical trial.[64] The results of an initial 4 infusion protocol were 45% of patients responding and 27% remitting, lower than the rates from many published trials of longer duration. These patients were followed for a year with no reported adverse effects or ketamine misuse. The most significant finding came from their follow up of a subset of 14 patients who received continuing maintenance infusions for periods varying from 14 to 126 weeks. Notably there were no reports of adverse side effects in this group – no cognitive decline, no delusional symptoms nor cystitis, no evidence of misuse.

Reports from other studies can be found in Chapters 9 and 10, examining such topics as the treatment of anxiety disorders, the management of suicidal thinking and clinical trials involving esketamine.

So what have we learned through the retrospectoscope? For the most part, early researchers were working either alone or in poorly funded positions, and it is only in recent years that the pace of investigation has quickened and the word spread outside the main research domains.

A good number of researchers from around the world have now established that ketamine given to treatment-resistant patients can:

1. rapidly lift depression after a single dose, although some may take longer to respond.
2. be effective given orally, sublingually, subcutaneously, intranasally, intramuscularly, and intravenously.
3. have longer lasting benefits following the use of multiple doses.

This chapter has given an overview of the work done so far. In the next, I will analyse more closely just how well ketamine works for depression.

References

1. Maia Szalavitz, 'Tackling Depression with Ketamine', *New Scientist* (Jan 2007).
2. Robert M. Berman, Angela Cappiello, Amit Anand, Dan A. Oren, George R. Heninger, Dennis S. Charney, and John H. Krystal, 'Antidepressant Effects of Ketamine in Depressed Patients', *Biological Psychiatry*, 47/4 (15 February 2000), 351–354.
3. A. Kudoh, Y. Takahira, H. Katagai, and T. Takazawa, 'Small-Dose Ketamine Improves the Postoperative State of Depressed Patients', *Anesthesia & Analgesia*, 95/1 (July 2002), 114–8.
4. Robert Ostroff, Marbiela Gonzales, Gerard Sanacora, 'Antidepressant Effect of Ketamine during ECT'. Am J Psychiatry. 2005 Jul;162(7):1385-6.
5. Graeme E. Correll and Graham E. Futter, 'Two Case Studies o f Patients with Major Depressive Disorder Given Low-Dose (Subanesthetic) Ketamine Infusions', *Pain Medicine*, 7/1 (2006).
6. Carlos A. Zarate Jr, Jaskaran B. Singh, Paul J. Carlson, Nancy E. Brutsche, Rezvan Ameli, David A. Luckenbaugh, Dennis S. Charney, Husseini K. Manji, 'A Randomized Trial of an N-methyl-D-aspartate Antagonist in Treatment-Resistant Major Depression', *Arch Gen Psychiatry*, 63 (2006), 856–864.
7. Michael Liebrenz, A. Borgeat, R. Leisinger, R. Stohler. 'Intravenous Ketamine Therapy in a Patient with a Treatment-Resistant Major Depression', *Swiss Med Weekly*, 137 (2007), 234–236.
8. M. Liebrenz, R. Stohler, A. Borgeat, 'Repeated intravenous ketamine therapy in a patient with treatment-resistant major depression', *World Journal of Biological Psychiatry*, 10/4 Pt 2 (2009), 640–3.
9. G. Paslakis M. Gilles, A. Meyer-Lindenberg and M. Deuschle. 'Oral Administration of the NMDA Receptor Antagonist S-Ketamine as Add-On Therapy of Depression: A Case Series', *Pharmacopsychiatry*.

10. Rebecca B. Price, Matthew K. Nock, Dennis S. Charney, and Sanjay J. Mathew, 'Effects of Intravenous Ketamine on Explicit and Implicit Measures of Suicidality in Treatment-Resistant Depression', *Biological Psychiatry*, 66/5 (1 September 2009), 522–526. DOI: 10.1016/j.biopsych.2009.04.029.

11. R. Paul, N. Schaaff, F. Padberg, H. J. Möller, T. Frodl, Department of Psychiatry and Psychotherapy, Ludwig-Maximilians-University, Munich, Germany. "Comparison of racemic and S-ketamine in treatment-resistant major depression." World J. Biol Psychiatry 2009; 10(3): 241-4.

12. F. Segmiller and C. Schüle, 'Repeated S-Ketamine Infusions in Treatment-Resistant Depression', *European Psychiatry*, 29/1 (2014), 1.

13. Scott A. Irwin and Alana Iglewicz, 'Oral Ketamine for the Rapid Treatment of Depression and Anxiety in Patients Receiving Hospice Care', *Journal of Palliative Medicine*, 13/7 (July 2010), 903–908. DOI: 10.1089/jpm.2010.9808.

14. S. J. Mathew, J. W. Murrough, M. aan het Rot, K. A. Collins, D. L. Reich, D. S. Charney, 'Riluzole for Relapse Prevention Following Intravenous Ketamine in Treatment-Resistant Depression: A Pilot Randomized, Placebo-Controlled Continuation Trial', *International Journal of Neuropsychopharmacology*, 13/1 (February 2010), 71–82. DOI: 10.1017/S1461145709000169.

15. Lobna Ibrahim, Nancy Diazgranados, Jose Franco-Chaves, Nancy Brutsche, Ioline D. Henter, Phillip Kronstein, Ruin Moaddel, Irving Wainer, David A. Luckenbaugh, Husseini K. Manji, and Carlos A. Zarate Jr, 'Course of Improvement in Depressive Symptoms to a Single Intravenous Infusion of Ketamine vs Add-on Riluzole: Results from a 4-Week, Double-Blind, Placebo-Controlled Study', *International Journal of Neuropsychopharmacology*, 37 (2012), 1526–1533. DOI: 10.1038/npp.2011.338. Published online 1 February 2012.

16. R. Kollmar, K. Markovic, N. Thürauf, H. Schmitt, and J. Kornhuber, 'Ketamine Followed by Memantine for the Treatment of Major Depression', *Australia & New Zealand Journal of Psychiatry*, 42/2 (February 2008): 170. DOI: 10.1080/00048670701787628.

17. M. aan het Rot, K. A. Collins, J. W. Murrough, A. M. Perez, D. L. Reich, D. S. Charney, S. J. Mathew, 'Safety and efficacy

of repeated-dose intravenous ketamine for treatment-resistant depression', *Biological Psychiatry*, 67/2 (15 January 2015), 139–45. DOI: 10.1016/j.biopsych.2009.08.038.

18. J. W. Murrough, A. M. Perez, S. Pillemer, J. Stern, M. K. Parides, M. aan het Rot, K. A. Collins, S. J. Mathew, D. S. Charney, D. V. Iosifescu, 'Rapid and Longer-Term Antidepressant Effects of Repeated Ketamine Infusions in Treatment-Resistant Major Depression', *Biological Psychiatry*, 74/4 (2013), 250–6.

19. Nancy Diazgranados, Lobna Ibrahim, Nancy E. Brutsche, Andrew Newberg, Phillip Kronstein, Sami Khalife, William A. Kammerer, Zenaide Quezado, David A. Luckenbaugh, Giacomo Salvadore, Rodrigo Machado-Vieira, Husseini K. Manji, and Carlos A. Zarate Jr, 'A Randomized Add-on Trial of an N-Methyl-D-Aspartate Antagonist in Treatment-Resistant Bipolar Depression', *Arch Gen Psychiatry*, 67/8 (August 2010), 793–802. DOI: 10.1001/archgenpsychiatry.2010.90.

20. C. A. Zarate Jr, N. E. Brutsche, L. Ibrahim, J. Franco-Chaves, N. Diazgranados, A. Cravchik, J. Selter, C. A. Marquardt, V. Liberty, D. A. Luckenbaugh, 'Replication of Ketamine's Antidepressant Efficacy in Bipolar Depression: A Randomized Controlled Add-On Trial', *Biological Psychiatry*, 71/11 (June 2012), 939–46. DOI: 10.1016/j.biopsych.2011.12.010.

21. Michael Messer, Irina V. Haller, Pamela Larson, Julia Pattison-Crisostomo, Charles E. Gessert, 'The Use of a Series of Ketamine Infusions in Two Patients with Treatment-Resistant Depression,' *Journal of Neuropsychiatry and Clinical Neurosciences*, 22 (2012), 442–444.

22. Claudia Grott Zanicotti, David Perez, and Paul Glue, 'Mood and pain responses to repeat dose intramuscular ketamine in a depressed patient with advanced cancer,' J Palliat Med. 2012 Apr;15(4):400-3.

23. P. Glue, A. Gulati, M. Le Nedelec, S. Duffull, 'Dose- and Exposure-Response to Ketamine in Depression Biological Psychiatry', *Biological Psychiatry*, 70/4 (15 August 2011), e9–10, author reply e11-2. DOI: 10.1016/j.biopsych.2010.11.

24. Cristina Cusin, George Q. Hilton, Andrew A. Nierenberg, Maurizio Fava, 'Long-Term Maintenance with Intramuscular Ketamine for Treatment-Resistant Bipolar II Depression',

American Journal of Psychiatry, 169 (1 August 2012), 868–869. DOI: 10.1176/appi.ajp.2012.12020219.

25. Demitri F. Papolos, Martin H. Teicher, Gianni L. Faedda, Patricia Murphy, Steven Mattis, 'Clinical Experience Using Intranasal Ketamine in the Treatment of Pediatric Bipolar Disorder/Fear of Harm Phenotype'. Journal of Affective disorders 147 (2013) 431-436.

26. Sarah M. Szymkowicz, Nora Finnegan, and Roman M. Daleb, 'A 12-Month Naturalistic Observation of Three Patients Receiving Repeat Intravenous Ketamine Infusions for Their Treatment-Resistant Depression'. The publisher's final edited version of this article is available at *Journal of Affective Disorders*.

27. McNulty, *International Journal of Pharmaceutical Compounding*, 16/5 (2012), 364–368.

28. P. Blier, D. Zigman, J. Blier, 'On the Safety and Benefits of Repeated Intravenous Injections of Ketamine for Depression', *Biological Psychiatry*, 72/4 (15 August 2012), e11–2. DOI: 10.1016/j.biopsych.2012.02.039.

29. H. Chilukuri, P. Dasari, J. S. Srinivas, 'Intramuscular Ketamine in Acute Depression: A Report on Two Cases', *Indian Journal of Psychiatry*, 55 (2013), 186–8.

30. Harihar Chilukuri, Narasimha Pothula Reddy, Ram Mohan Pathapati, Arkalgud Nagesha Manu, Sharada Jollu, and Ahammed Basha Shaik, 'Acute Antidepressant Effects of Intramuscular versus Intravenous Ketamine', *Indian Journal of Psychological Medicine*, 36/1 (January–March 2014): 71–76. DOI: 10.4103/0253-7176.127258.

31. S. A. Irwin, A. Iglewicz, R. A. Nelesen, J. Y. Lo, C. H. Carr, S. D. Romero, L. S. Lloyd, 'Daily Oral Ketamine for the Treatment of Depression and Anxiety in Patients Receiving Hospice Care: A 28-Day Open-Label Proof-of-Concept Trial'.

32. A. Iglewicz, K. Morrison, R. A. Nelesen, T. Zhan, B. Iglewicz, N. Fairman, J. M. Hirst, S. A. Irwin, 'Ketamine for the Treatment of Depression in Patients Receiving Hospice Care: A Retrospective Medical Record Review of Thirty-One Cases', *Psychosomatics*, 56/4 (July–August 2015), 329-37. DOI: 10.1016/j.psym.2014.05.005.

33. Messer, M. Haller, I. 'Maintenance Ketamine Treatment Produces Long-Term Recovery from Depression', *Primary Psychiatry* (21 May 2013).
34. Posted by 'Foreigner' on the Bluelight's ketamine forum 2013.
35. James W. Murrough, Dan V. Iosifescu, Lee C. Chang, Rayan K. Al Jurdi, Charles E. Green, Andrew M. Perez, Syed Iqbal, Sarah Pillemer, Alexandra Foulkes, Asim Shah, Dennis S. Charney, 'Antidepressant Efficacy of Ketamine in Treatment-Resistant Major Depression: A Two-Site Randomized Controlled Trial', *American Journal of Psychiatry*, 170 (2013), 1134–1142.
36. Keith G. Rasmussen, Timothy W. Lineberry, Christine W. Galardy, Simon Kung, Maria I. Lapid, Brian A. Palmer, Matthew J. Ritter, Kathryn M. Schak, Christopher L. Sola, Allison J. Hanson, and Mark A. Frye, 'Serial Infusions of Low-Dose Ketamine for Major Depression', *Journal of Psychopharmacology*, 27/5,(2103), 444–450.
37. Diogo R. Lara, Luisa W. Bisol, and Luciano R. Munari, 'Antidepressant, Mood Stabilizing and Procognitive Effects of Very Low Dose Sublingual Ketamine in Refractory Unipolar and Bipolar Depression', *International Journal of Neuropsychopharmacology*, 16 (2013), 2111–2117. DOI: 10.1017/S1461145713000485.
38. John Gever, 'Ketamine Works in OCD, Stubborn Depression', *MedPage Today*,. (2013)
39. Kyle A. B. Lapidus, Cara F. Levitch, Andrew M. Perez, Jess W. Brallier, Michael K. Parides, Laili Soleimani, Adriana Feder, Dan V. Iosifescu, Dennis S. Charney, James W. Murrough *Journal of Affective Disorders*, 147/0 (May 2013), 416–420. DOI: http://dx.doi.org/10.1016/j.biopsych.2014.03.026.
40. Jaskaran Singh, 'A Double-Blind, Randomized, Placebo-Controlled, Parallel Group, Dose Frequency Study of Intravenous Ketamine in Patients with Treatment-Resistant Depression', poster session 1, Janssen Research and Development, LLC, Tuesday, 17 June 2014.
41. Peter R. Diamond, Andrew D. Farmery, Stephanie Atkinson, Jag Haldar, Nicola Williams, Phil J. Cowen, John R. Geddes, and Rupert McShane, 'Ketamine Infusions for Treatment Resistant Depression: A Series of 28 Patients Treated Weekly or Twice

Weekly in an ECT Clinic', *Journal of Psychopharmacology* (2014), 1–9. DOI: 10.1177/0269881114527361.

42. Cathy (21 May 2014). <medchat.com>.

43. Patricia Clark, 'Treatment-Refractory Depression: A Case of Successful Treatment with Intranasal Ketamine 10%', *Annals of Clinical Psychiatry*, 26/1 (2014), e10.

44. Veronica Gálvez, Emily O'Keefe, Laura Cotiga, John Leyden, Simon Harper, Paul Glue, Philip B. Mitchell, Andrew A. Somogyi, Amanda DeLory, Colleen K. Loo, 'Long-Lasting Effects of a Single Subcutaneous Dose of Ketamine for Treating Melancholic Depression: A Case Report', *Biological Psychiatry* (2014). <http://dx.doi.org/10.1016/j.biopsych.2013.12.010>.

45. Nguyen, L., Marshalek, P. J., Weaver, C. B., Cramer, K. J., Pollard, S. E., & Matsumoto, R. R. (2015). Off-label use of transmucosal ketamine as a rapid-acting antidepressant: a retrospective chart review. Neuropsychiatric Disease and Treatment, 11, 2667-2673. doi: 10.2147/NDT.S88569

46. Hu, Y. D., Sha, S., Shi, H., Xue, Y., Tian, T. F., Ma, X., . . . Chiu, H. F. K. (2016). Single i.v. ketamine augmentation of newly initiated escitalopram for major depression: Results from a randomized, placebo-controlled 4-week study. Psychological Medicine, 46(3), 623-635. doi: 10.1017/S0033291715002159

47. Zhang et al. Journal International Psychiatry 2018-02 Liaocheng Fourth Peoples Hospital.

48. Domani, Y., Bleich-Cohen, M., Stoppelman, N., Tarrasch, R., Hendler, T., Meidan, R., . . . Sharon, H. (2016). Oral ketamine for treatment resistant major depression; A double blind randomized controlled trial. European Psychiatry, 33, S523. doi: 10.1016/j.eurpsy.2016.01.1528

49. Jafarinia, M., Afarideh, M., Tafakhori, A., Arbabi, M., Ghajar, A., Noorbala, A. A., . . . Akhondzadeh, S. (2016). Efficacy and safety of oral ketamine versus diclofenac to alleviate mild to moderate depression in chronic pain patients: A double-blind, randomized, controlled trial. Journal of Affective Disorders, 204, 1-8. doi: 10.1016/j.jad.2016.05.076

50. Lenze, E. J., Farber, N. B., Kharasch, E., Schweiger, J., Yingling, M., Olney, J., & Newcomer, J. W. (2016). Ninety-six hour ketamine infusion with co-administered clonidine for treatment-resistant

depression: a pilot randomized controlled trial. The world journal of biological psychiatry : the official journal of the World Federation of Societies of Biological Psychiatry, 17(3), 230-238. doi: 10.3109/15622975.2016.1142607

51. Cohen, I. V., Makunts, T., Atayee, R., & Abagyan, R. (2017). Population scale data reveals the antidepressant effects of ketamine and other therapeutics approved for non-psychiatric indications. Scientific Reports, 7(1), 1450. doi: 10.1038/s41598-017-01590-x

52. George, D., Gálvez, V., Martin, D., Kumar, D., Leyden, J., Hadzi-Pavlovic, D., . . . Loo, C. K. (2017). Pilot Randomized Controlled Trial of Titrated Subcutaneous Ketamine in Older Patients with Treatment-Resistant Depression. The American Journal of Geriatric Psychiatry, 25(11), 1199-1209. doi: https://doi.org/10.1016/j.jagp.2017.06.007

53. Medeiros da Frota Ribeiro, C., & Riva-Posse, P. (2017). Use of Ketamine in Elderly Patients with Treatment-Resistant Depression. Current Psychiatry Reports, 19(12), 107. doi: 10.1007/s11920-017-0855-x

54. Al Shirawi, M. I., Kennedy, S. H., Ho, K. T., Byrne, R., & Downar, J. (2017). Oral Ketamine in Treatment-Resistant Depression: A Clinical Effectiveness Case Series. Journal of Clinical Psychopharmacology, 37(4), 464-467. doi: 10.1097/JCP.0000000000000717

55. Cusin, C., Ionescu, D. F., Pavone, K. J., Akeju, O., Cassano, P., Taylor, N., . . . Fava, M. (2016). Ketamine augmentation for outpatients with treatment-resistant depression: Preliminary evidence for two-step intravenous dose escalation. Australian & New Zealand Journal of Psychiatry, 51(1), 55-64. doi: 10.1177/0004867416631828

56. Papakostas et al. "IV ketamine proves superior to active placebo in low, high doses." Whitney McKnight, Clinical Psychiatry News 2017.

57. Arabzadeh, S., Hakkikazazi, E., Shahmansouri, N., Tafakhori, A., Ghajar, A., Jafarinia, M., & Akhondzadeh, S. (2018). Does oral administration of ketamine accelerate response to treatment in major depressive disorder? Results of a double-blind controlled trial. Journal of Affective Disorders, 235, 236-241. doi: 10.1016/j.jad.2018.02.056

58. Papolos, D., Frei, M., Rossignol, D., Mattis, S., Hernandez-Garcia, L. C., & Teicher, M. H. (2018). Clinical experience using intranasal ketamine in the longitudinal treatment of juvenile bipolar disorder with fear of harm phenotype. Journal of Affective Disorders, 225, 545-551. doi: 10.1016/j.jad.2017.08.081

59. Cullen, K. R., Amatya, P., Roback, M. G., Albott, C. S., Westlund Schreiner, M., Ren, Y., . . . Klimes-Dougan, B. (2018). Intravenous Ketamine for Adolescents with Treatment-Resistant Depression: An Open-Label Study. Journal of Child and Adolescent Psychopharmacology. doi: 10.1089/cap.2018.0030

60. Hartberg, J., Garrett-Walcott, S., & De Gioannis, A. (2018). Impact of oral ketamine augmentation on hospital admissions in treatment-resistant depression and PTSD: a retrospective study. Psychopharmacology, 235(2), 393-398. doi: 10.1007/s00213-017-4786-3

61. Gamble, J. J., Bi, H., Bowen, R., Weisgerber, G., Sanjanwala, R., Prasad, R., & Balbuena, L. (2018). Ketamine-based anesthesia improves electroconvulsive therapy outcomes: a randomized-controlled study. Canadian Journal of Anesthesia/Journal canadien d'anesthésie, 65(6), 636-646. doi: 10.1007/s12630-018-1088-0

62. Ghasemi, M., Kazemi, M. H., Yoosefi, A., Ghasemi, A., Paragomi, P., Amini, H., & Afzali, M. H. (2014). Rapid antidepressant effects of repeated doses of ketamine compared with electroconvulsive therapy in hospitalized patients with major depressive disorder. Psychiatry Research, 215(2), 355-361. doi: https://doi.org/10.1016/j.psychres.2013.12.008

63. Albott, C. S., Lim, K. O., Forbes, M. K., Grabowski, J. G., Batres-Y-Carr, T. M., Shiroma, P. R., . . . Wels, J. (2018). Efficacy, safety, and durability of repeated ketamine infusions for comorbid posttraumatic stress disorder and treatment-resistant depression. Journal of Clinical Psychiatry, 79(3). doi: 10.4088/JCP.17m11634

64. Miriam Davis et al. "Treatment-resistant mood disorders: long-term ketamine found safe, modestly effective." J Clinical Psychiatry, 26 Jul 2018.

Chapter 4

Does It Work?

In the last chapter, I outlined the research into the use of ketamine for treatment-resistant depression conducted over the last 18 years. Positive findings have come from a series of trials, ranging from single-case reports to randomised, double-blind, placebo-controlled studies. And ketamine has proved effective for patients when given through a variety of routes ranging from oral to intravenous infusions.

Most of the early studies focused on establishing that a single dose of ketamine can produce rapid improvement which for some can last for weeks.

We can be most confident about the validity of results from studies that recruit large numbers of patients (more than 100) suffering from similar conditions and using reliable placebos. Studies meeting these criteria have been rare, and for financial reasons, we are unlikely to see many in the future. However, there is a statistical strategy used in this situation, which involves combining the results of a number of small trials and, in effect, creating one large trial and then analysing the outcomes.

This is known as a meta-analysis, and in the past two years, there have been a number published on the treatment of depression with ketamine. The following are their conclusions, and the references at the end of this chapter will give you more detailed information. I have also included comments from recent comprehensive reviews of the evidence concerning ketamine in the treatment of depression.

The following is the review of Katalinic et al. in 2013:[1]

> Overall, while almost all studies have found significant anti-depressant effects with ketamine administration, it is clear that not all patients respond. With the increasing number of studies finding rapid and substantial effects in a proportion of their patients, research should begin to focus on identifying predictors of response. Moreover, maintenance of these effects continues to be a major limitation. Of the studies that followed participants until relapse, about one-third reported relapse within 3 days, one-third reported relapse in about a week, and one-third reported relapse between 20 and 40 days. Generally, it appears that frequent, repeated infusions (in a model similar to an ECT course) may prolong the period of remission. While pretreatment with lamotrigine and riluzole were found to be unsuccessful in significantly prolonging remission, one case study found positive results with memantine.

The following is the meta-analysis of Fond et al. in 2014:[2]

> The present meta-analysis confirms ketamine's efficacy in depressive disorders in non-ECT studies, as well as in ECT studies. The results of this first meta-analysis are encouraging, and further studies are warranted to detail efficacy in bipolar disorders and other specific depressed populations. Middle and long-term efficacy and safety have yet to be explored. Extrapolation should be cautious: Patients included had no history of psychotic episodes and no history of alcohol or substance use disorders, which is not representative of all the depressed patients that may benefit from this therapy.

The following is the meta-analysis of McGirr et al. in 2014:[3]

> Our meta-analysis suggests that single administrations of ketamine are efficacious in the rapid treatment of unipolar and bipolar depression. Additional research is required

to determine optimal dosing schedules, route, treatment schedules, and the potential efficacy of other glutamatergic agents.

The following is the meta-analysis of Caddy et al. in 2014:[4]

In total, 22 RCTs [randomised controlled trials] and non-RCTs were identified that investigated the potential role of ketamine as an antidepressant in MDD and BPAD, totalling 629 participants. Ketamine infusion resulted in a rapid antidepressant effect in the vast majority of the presented studies, either administered alone, with an augmenter, or in combination with ECT. Furthermore, several recent studies demonstrated a rapid antisuicidal effect that was independent of antidepressant response. High response rates were documented in many studies, with three of the included RCTs recording a 71–79% response rate at 24 hours post-ketamine infusion. This is a considerable response rate to be observed at this early time point, certainly when compared with traditional monoaminergic [affecting single receptors, usually serotonin] antidepressants wherein response rates of 65% following 6–8 weeks of treatment are notable.

The following is the review of Ryan et al. in 2014:[5]

Thorough review of the literature utilising ketamine for treatment-refractory depression reveals rapid onset of action in the first several hours, often lasting several days to a week, after a single infusion. We acknowledge a common criticism raised about the limited time frame of efficacy from a single dose of ketamine, however this does not distinguish it from any other treatment of depression, including psychotherapy, medication, or ECT. Furthermore, multiple dosing studies and alternate routes of administration have safely and successfully extended the antidepressant benefit of ketamine, with select cases demonstrating maintenance for nearly a year. These findings are all the more impressive when viewed from the perspective of an already treatment-resistant population. While the existing paradigm of 40-minute IV infusions has proven limitedly effective, much less resource intensive protocols such as intranasal, intramuscular, oral, and subcutaneous methods of administration represent a potential revolution in the use of ketamine. These routes of administration have the advantage of expanding ketamine research to the outpatient setting. We did not find evidence of serious neurocognitive adverse effects in clinical use, in contrast to what has been reported with ketamine abuse. This is an area in which ketamine may distinguish itself from ECT as an alternative for TRD. Similarly, we did not find evidence of LUTS [lower urinary tract symptoms] but this has not been systematically investigated. The frequency and seriousness of LUTS in the abuse population makes it an important adverse effect to monitor in future long-term studies. Dissociative effects are common, time limited, generally well tolerated and appear to subside in intensity with repeat dosing. These and other unique effects distinguish it from currently used monoaminergic antidepressants and warrant further study in terms of their ability to advance understanding of depression and its treatment. Significant hemodynamic effects requiring intervention are possible but uncommon, and do require careful monitoring. Potential contraindications do exist, including psychosis, abuse liability, and hemodynamic instability, but with care in patient selection unwanted outcomes can be minimised. Ketamine is clearly a very promising agent. While we must urge caution in wide spread clinical application before further research is completed, our review of the risks and benefits supports its use in carefully selected cases who have not benefited from other treatments.

Ido Efrati wrote in 2015:[6]

'We have recently been witnessing a boom of studies on the subject of ketamine,' said Dr Revital Amiaz, director of the Clinic for Depression, Anxiety and Electroconvulsive Treatment at the Sheba Medical Centre, Tel Hashomer. 'We're talking about some 20 studies, and another three meta-analyses that combine and summarise the results of the most recent trials. This information already sums up trials conducted on about 800 patients. And the results are becoming increasingly convincing.'

The following is the meta-analysis of Lee et al. in 2015:[7]

The large and statistically significant effect of ketamine on depressive symptoms supports a promising, new and effective pharmacotherapy with rapid onset, high efficacy and good tolerability.

The following is the meta-analysis of Coyle and Laws in 2015:[8]

Single ketamine infusions elicit a significant antidepressant effect from 4 h to 7 days; the small number of studies at 12–14 days post infusion failed to reach significance. Results suggest a discrepancy in peak response time depending upon primary diagnosis—24 h for MDD and 7 days for BD. The majority of published studies have used pre-post comparison; further placebo-controlled studies would help to clarify the effect of ketamine over time.

Michael Bloch's meta-analysis in 2015 was reported on *Bipolar News* online:[9]

Ketamine, an anaesthetic sometimes used intravenously in the treatment of depression, can bring about rapid onset of antidepressant effects. A new meta-analysis by researcher Michael Bloch and colleagues presented at a recent conference showed that ketamine's maximum antidepressant effects occur within one day of administration and its effects remain significant (compared to control conditions) one week following infusion. Ketamine's effects were diminished in patients taking other medications. There was a trend for better response in patients with bipolar disorder than with unipolar disorder.

Bloch and colleagues analysed eight earlier studies including a total of 180 participants. In each study ketamine had been compared to a control condition, either an infusion of saline solution or of midazolam, which mimics ketamine's sensory effects but does not have antidepressant effects. The researchers are calling for more meta-analyses of ketamine studies to determine which patients respond best to ketamine and how to sustain Ketamine's effects.

This meta-analysis from 2016 published by Yu Han et al examined 9 double-blind randomised, placebo controlled studies involving 368 patients.[11] They looked at results at 24 hours, 72 hours and 7 days post infusion finding significant benefits for the ketamine group compared to placebo. At 24 hours post-infusion the response rate for the ketamine group was 52% and the remission rate was 21%, at 72 hours the response rate was 48% and remission rate was 24% and at 7 days the response rate was 40% and remission rate 26%.

Half the patients studied had treatment-resistant depression, 7 of the 9 placebos used in the trials were saline.

The treatment was well tolerated overall.

In a review in 2017 Kraus et al assessed the evidence concerning ketamine's efficacy in both unipolar and bipolar depression.[12] They evaluated 19 studies, 12 on unipolar and 7 on bipolar depression, with the majority using the intravenous route and the remainder intranasal administration.

They noted response rates of up to 88% with an average effect of 61% and mild side effects particularly compared to ECT, which is another option for these patients.

They concluded, "After a single infusion, strong antidepressant effects could be observed after several hours post-infusion lasting for 7–14 days. Although rates of depressive relapse vary between trials, these occur in up to 90% of patients within 2 weeks after treatment. Taken together, existing evidence suggests that ketamine may act as a potent and rapid antidepressant with anti-suicidal action in acute suicidal crises, as well as treatment in highly resistant forms of depression."

From Mexico City Rodrigo Perez-Esparza stated in his review in 2018 that ketamine's positives lay in its demonstrated efficacy in both major depression and bipolar disorder, in its rapid action, its ability to bring about prolonged responses and remissions, the rapid reduction of suicidality often seen and the transitory mild side effects.[13]

The current concerns included possible long-term side effects e.g. cystitis, the potential for misuse, the increasing off-label use that has been occurring and the insufficient long-term safety and efficacy data.

There is now abundant evidence of the short-term efficacy and safety of ketamine administered through a variety of routes. The crucial evidence concerning the efficacy of maintenance therapy, which most patients require, is now coming from two sources – the researchers from Janssen who are accumulating long-term data on treatment with intranasal esketamine [see Chapter 10] and the information coming from physicians who are treating growing numbers of people over extended time periods. [See Chapters 6,7]

To summarise, at all levels of evidence from the anecdotal to the randomised controlled trials, ketamine is efficacious for many patients with treatment-resistant depression. Actual results vary according to illness-severity, dose, setting, and the mode of administration. It appears that those with 'pure', less-severe episodes of depression respond more quickly at lower doses and for longer. For some, ketamine may give lasting benefit. Many will gain at least temporary relief, and all will appreciate the opportunity to try a new treatment for a debilitating illness.

Patients gave these accounts on the Ketamine Advocacy Network:[10]
Patient R. S. (male, suffered for 30 years) said, 'I can't believe the huge difference these tiny gains have made in my life. I thought ketamine would give me an instant sense of wellbeing that I could feel

in my gut, and then I would use it like a weapon to conquer the world and do the things I want. But it actually worked the other way around. Ketamine gave me the ability to do a bunch of small routine things that I could never do before, and together they've made my entire life easier. The sense of wellbeing sneaked up on me. Instead of coming directly from the infusions like I expected, it came from doing all these new things that ketamine has freed me to do.'

Patient S. P. (female, suffered 20 years) said, I thought I'd be blasted with relief. Like from a fire hose. I squinched my eyes and tensed up waiting for the blast. The longer I waited the more tense I got. It distracted me from the pool of relief that formed silently under my feet over the course of three infusions. I didn't notice it until I was completely soaked from the bottom up. Frankly I was disappointed because I imagined the blast would be so awesome. But once I realised I was drenched in relief and was actually functioning and living life again, the blast seemed pointless.'

References

1. Natalie Katalinic, Rosalyn Lai, Andrew Somogyi, Philip B. Mitchell, Paul Glue, and Colleen K. Loo, 'Ketamine as a New Treatment for Depression: A Review of Its Efficacy and Adverse Effects', *Australia & New Zealand Journal of Psychiatry* (9 May 2013). DOI: 10.1177/0004867413486842.

2. Guillaume Fond, Anderson Loundou, Corentin Rabu, Alexandra Macgregor, Christophe Lançon, Marie Brittner, Jean-Arthur Micoulaud-Franchi, Richeiri R, Courtet F, Abbar m, Roger M, Leboyer M, Boyer L, 'Ketamine Administration in Depressive Disorders: A Systematic Review and Meta-Analysis', *Psychopharmacology*. DOI: 10.1007/s00213-014-3664-.

3. A. McGirr, M.T.Berlim, D.J. Bond, M.P. Fleck, L.N. Yatham and R.W. Lam. 'A Systematic Review and Meta-Analysis of Randomized, Double-Blind, Placebo-Controlled Trials of Ketamine in the Rapid Treatment of Major Depressive Episodes', *Psychological Medicine* (July 2014). DOI: 10.1017/S0033291714001603.

4. Caroline Caddy, Giovanni Giaroli, Thomas P. White, Sukhwinder S. Shergill, and Derek K. Tracy, 'Ketamine as the Prototype

Glutamatergic Antidepressant: Pharmacodynamic Actions, and a Systematic Review and Meta-Analysis of Efficacy', *Therapeutic Advances in Psychopharmacology*, 4/2 (April 2014), 75–99. DOI: 10.1177/2045125313507739.

5. Wesley C. Ryan, Cole J. Marta, and Ralph J. Koek, 'Ketamine and Depression: A Review', *International Journal of Transpersonal Studies*, 33/2 (2014), 40–74.

6. Ido Efrati, 'Ketamine Praised for Speedily Alleviating Depression' ('Haaretz', January 26, 2015).

7. E. E. Lee, M. P. Della Selva, A. Liu, S. Himelhoch, 'Ketamine as a Novel Treatment for Major Depressive Disorder and Bipolar Depression: A Systematic Review and Quantitative Meta-Analysis', *General Hospital Psychiatry*, 37/2 (March–April 2015), 178–84. DOI: 10.1016/j.genhosppsych.2015.01.003.

8. C. M. Coyle and K. R. Laws, 'The Use of Ketamine as an Antidepressant: A Systematic Review and Meta-Analysis', Human Psychopharmacology Clinical and Experimental. DOI: 10.1002/hup.2475.

9. 'Meta-Analysis Shows Effectiveness of Ketamine for Bipolar and Unipolar Depression', *Bipolar News* (22 April 2015).

10. Ketamine Advocacy Network. <www.ketamineadvocacynetwork.org>.

11. Han, Y., Chen, J., Zou, D., Zheng, P., Li, Q., Wang, H., . . . Xie, P. (2016). Efficacy of ketamine in the rapid treatment of major depressive disorder: a meta-analysis of randomized, double-blind, placebo-controlled studies. Neuropsychiatric Disease and Treatment, 12, 2859-2867. doi: 10.2147/NDT.S117146

12. Kraus, C., Rabl, U., Vanicek, T., Carlberg, L., Popovic, A., Spies, M., . . . Kasper, S. (2017). Administration of ketamine for unipolar and bipolar depression. International Journal of Psychiatry in Clinical Practice, 21(1), 2-12. doi: 10.1080/13651501.2016.1254802

13. Pérez-Esparza, R. (2018). Ketamine for Treatment-Resistant Depression: a New Advocate. Revista De Investigacion Clinica; Organo Del Hospital De Enfermedades De La Nutricion, 70(2), 65-67. doi: 10.24875/RIC.18002501

Chapter 5

How Does It Work?

We are always seeking simple answers to complex problems—and they're nearly always wrong.[1]

Before looking at the ways ketamine may work to relieve a depressive illness, we should look a little more deeply into what we are actually treating.

Feelings of depression are as old as life itself. As a response to loss, we experience the sensations of aloneness, joylessness, helplessness, hopelessness, and despair. However, when these feelings of depression persist for weeks and months on end and are joined by other changes (such as problems with sleep, appetite, energy, concentration, and negative patterns of thought), our whole being, body, mind, and spirit become diminished, and there is a clear reduction in our ability to function in everyday life. This is when the diagnosis of a depressive illness is made.

A depressive illness is not a 'disease,' that being a condition with a known cause, a clear pathology, and a response to a specific treatment. In our current state of knowledge, a depressive illness is more like a fever, a collection of symptoms and signs indicating a disorder and arising from a range of different causes. We are still in the early stages of the process of understanding the vulnerabilities, the triggers, the areas of the brain affected, and the best ways of promoting healing.

What we have learned is that effective treatment first requires the formation of a strong alliance between doctor and patient and then a thorough assessment of the problem and immediate measures to improve sleep, exercise levels, and nutrition as well as reduction of any substance misuse. In the longer term, the task is to help people change negative beliefs and behaviours and to address any past trauma. In addition to this, we have medications that help deal with the disconnections that occur on the electrochemical level.

In this context, with ketamine being just one component of an overall treatment plan, we can examine what we have learned so far about where and how it acts on the brain.

This chapter uses a number of scientific terms which refer to the structure and function of brain areas affected by ketamine. They are described in the following glossary:

- *neurone* —This is a cell of the nervous system. Neurones typically consist of a cell body, which contains a nucleus and receives incoming nerve impulses through dendrites, and an axon, which carries impulses away from the cell body.
- *synapse*—This is a specialised junction at which a neurone communicates with a target cell. At a synapse, a neurone releases a chemical transmitter that diffuses across a small gap and activates special sites called receptors on the target cell. The target cell may be another neurone or a specialised region of a muscle or secretory cell. Neurones can also communicate through direct electrical connections.
- *neurotransmitters*—These are chemicals that transmit signals across a synapse from one neurone to another 'target' neurone. Glutamate is thought to be the most important neurotransmitter in the brain. The majority of excitatory neurones in the central nervous system are glutamergic, and over half of all brain synapses release this agent. Through its role in synaptic plasticity, glutamate is involved in cognitive functions, such as learning and memory.
- *NMDA receptor*—The N-methyl-D-aspartate receptor is a glutamate receptor found in nerve cells. It is activated when glutamate and glycine bind to it, and when activated, it allows positively charged ions to flow through the cell membrane.
- *mTOR*—The mammalian target of rapamycin (mTOR) signalling pathway integrates both intracellular and extracellular signals and serves as a central regulator of cell metabolism, growth, proliferation, and survival.

- *BDNF*—The BDNF gene produces brain-derived neurotrophic factor, a protein found in the brain and spinal cord. This protein promotes the survival of neurones by playing a role in the growth, maturation, and maintenance of these cells. In the brain, the BDNF protein is active at the connections between nerve cells (synapses), where cell-to-cell communication occurs. The synapses can change and adapt over time in response to experience, a characteristic called synaptic plasticity. The BDNF protein helps regulate synaptic plasticity, which is important for learning and memory.
- *epigenetic*—This refers to external modifications to DNA that turn genes 'on' or 'off'. These modifications do not change the DNA sequence.
- *hippocampus*—Latin for *seahorse*, the hippocampus is named for its shape. It is part of a system that directs many bodily functions—the *limbic system*. This system is located in the brain's medial temporal lobe, near the centre of the brain. The hippocampus is involved in the storage of long-term memory, which includes all past knowledge and experiences. In particular, the hippocampus plays a major role in declarative memory, the type of memory involving things that can be purposely recalled, such as facts or events.
- *prefrontal cortex*—This brain region contributes to planning, personality expression, decision-making, and moderating social behaviour.

Previous theories concerning the action of the traditional antidepressants focused on two chemical messengers in the brain, serotonin and noradrenaline. They posited that reductions in levels of these compounds were associated with depression and that taking antidepressants restored this balance. However, the long-time delay to the lifting of mood was puzzling as the chemical changes in the brain after taking antidepressants occurred quickly. In the next development, it was discovered that, two-three weeks after antidepressant administration, there was an increase in the number of new nerve cells formed in specific brain areas (e.g. the hippocampus) and that this occurred not only as a consequence of antidepressant use but also with other effective treatments, such as psychotherapy, exercise, and ECT.

However, the brain has relatively small numbers of serotonin and noradrenaline neurones, around 50,000 for noradrenaline and 500,000 for serotonin out of a total of 85 billion, so they are important, but they are not the main players in brain signalling. By contrast, the glutamate system on which ketamine primarily acts is the major excitatory neurotransmitter system in the brain.

In 2010 research conducted by Duman and associates at Yale University revealed that administering ketamine to rats led to increased growth and function in dendritic spine synapses in the prefrontal cortex.[2]

Duman believes that ketamine rapidly increases the communication among existing neurones by creating these new connections. This is a quicker process than waiting for new neurones to form, and it accomplishes the same goal of enhancing brain circuit activity. This increase in neuronal connectivity is thought to relieve depression.[2a]

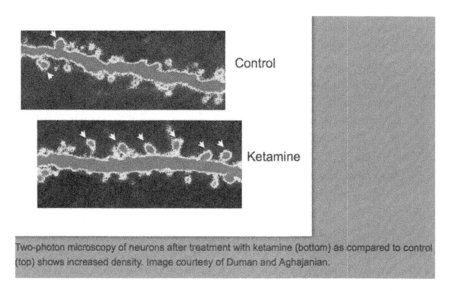

Two-photon microscopy of neurons after treatment with ketamine (bottom) as compared to control (top) shows increased density. Image courtesy of Duman and Aghajanian.

To explore the action of ketamine on NMDA receptors in a little more depth, the following study examines the make-up and function of the NMDA receptor in mice:

> Neurones communicate with one another by releasing chemicals known as neurotransmitters which transfer information by binding to receptor proteins on the surface of other neurones. Drugs such as ketamine also bind to these

receptors. Ketamine works by blocking a specific receptor called the n-methyl d-aspartate (NMDA) receptor, but how this produces antidepressant effects is not fully understood.

The NMDA receptor is actually formed from a combination of individual protein subunits, including one called GluN2B. Now, **Oliver Miller, Lingling Yang and colleagues** have created mice that lack receptors containing these GluN2B subunits in neurones in their neocortex, including the prefrontal cortex, a brain region involved in complex mental processes such as decision-making. This allowed Miller, Yang and colleagues to discover that when neurotransmitter glutamate binds to GluN2B-containing NMDA receptors, it limits the production of certain proteins that make it easier for signals to be transmitted between neurones. Suppressing the synthesis of these proteins too much may cause depressive effects by reducing communication between the neurones in the prefrontal cortex.

Both mice lacking GluN2B-containing receptors in their cortical neurones and normal mice treated with ketamine showed a reduced amount of depressive-like behaviour. This evidence supports Miller, Yang et al.'s theory that by blocking these NMDA receptors, ketamine restricts their activation. This restores normal levels of protein synthesis, improves communication between neurones in the cortex, and reduces depression.

Understanding how ketamine works to alleviate depression is an important step towards developing it into a safe and effective treatment. Further research is also required to determine the conditions that cause overactivation of the GluN2B-containing NMDA receptors.[4]

One of the likely ways that ketamine brings about such rapid improvement in depressive symptoms comes from its effect on signalling pathways.

In preclinical models of despair in rats, ketamine activates the mammalian target of rapamycin (mTOR), which is a critical hub of cellular growth and proliferation. Ketamine increased mTOR phosphorylation and other downstream molecular targets critical for transcriptional activation within one hour of administration. Twenty four hours following ketamine exposure, greater numbers of mature dendritic spines were observed. These molecular and cellular effects were lost if the rodent was pre-treated with rapamycin, an mTOR antagonist. Interestingly, rapid antidepressant-like behaviours in rodents were only observed following treatment with low doses (10–20 mg/kg) as opposed to higher anaesthetic doses (80 mg/kg), suggesting an inverted 'U' dose-effect relationship. In all, these findings suggest that mTOR activation is necessary for ketamine's rapid-acting antidepressant effects in a rodent model of despair, which may occur through BDNF.[5]

One hypothesis is that chronic stress in vulnerable people leads to loss of neurotropic cell-protecting factors (e.g. BDNF), which in turn leads to reversible structural changes manifested by a loss of connections and nerve cell atrophy.

Increasing BDNF levels gives rise to new neurones with the right connections, more branches (arborisation), more protrusions and more synapses.

Infusing BDNF into rat brains causes a rapid antidepressant effect, whereas blocking BDNF blocks ketamine's rapid antidepressant effect. Conventional antidepressants by contrast have only slow and modest effects on BDNF levels.

At another level, researchers are examining how communication between brain areas is affected by stress.

Studies in animals and then in humans have shown that prefrontal circuits are taken "off-line" during stress exposure. With prolonged stress exposure, there are additional architectural changes, such as loss of spines and dendrites in those circuits that provide top-down regulation, and increased dendritic arborisation in those circuits that drive the stress response.[6]

Specific areas of the prefrontal cortex have been shown to function differently in depression. The following study links ketamine's antidepressant activity to a specific part of this cortex:

> Ketamine produces rapid and sustained antidepressant actions in depressed patients, but the precise cellular mechanisms underlying these effects have not been identified. Here we determined if modulation of neuronal activity in the infralimbic prefrontal cortex (IL-PFC) underlies the antidepressant and anxiolytic actions of ketamine. We found that neuronal inactivation of the IL-PFC completely blocked the antidepressant and anxiolytic effects of systemic ketamine in rodent models and that ketamine microinfusion into IL-PFC reproduced these behavioural actions of systemic ketamine. We also found that optogenetic stimulation of the IL-PFC [in optogenetics, a molecule that causes neuronal activation in response to light of a particular wavelength is inserted into specific cells—in this case, by means of a customised virus—and these neurones can then be activated selectively with pulsating light] produced rapid and long-lasting antidepressant and anxiolytic effects and that these effects are associated with increased number and function of spine synapses of layer V pyramidal neurones. The results demonstrate that ketamine infusions or optogenetic stimulation of IL-PFC are sufficient to produce long-lasting antidepressant behavioural and synaptic responses similar to the effects of systemic ketamine administration.[7]

Recently it has become possible to measure the strength of connections between different brain areas affected by depression.

> Major depressive disorder was characterised by hypoconnectivity within the frontoparietal network, a set of regions involved in cognitive control of attention and emotion regulation, and hypoconnectivity between frontoparietal systems and parietal regions of the dorsal attention network involved in attending to the external environment. Major depressive disorder was also associated

with hyperconnectivity within the default network, a network believed to support internally oriented and self-referential thought, and hyperconnectivity between frontoparietal control systems and regions of the default network. Finally, the MDD groups exhibited hypoconnectivity between neural systems involved in processing emotion or salience and midline cortical regions that may mediate top-down regulation of such functions.

Conclusions and Relevance

Reduced connectivity within frontoparietal control systems and imbalanced connectivity between control systems and networks involved in internal or external attention may reflect depressive biases toward internal thoughts at the cost of engaging with the external world. Meanwhile, altered connectivity between neural systems involved in cognitive control and those that support salience or emotion processing may relate to deficits regulating mood. These findings provide an empirical foundation for a neurocognitive model in which network dysfunction underlies core cognitive and affective abnormalities in depression.[8]

The effects of ketamine on the brain circuits in monkeys have been recently reported.

Abstract

Background:

Ketamine is a highly attractive candidate for developing fast-onset antidepressant agents; however, the relevant brain circuits that underlie sustained, efficacious antidepressant effects remain largely unknown.

Methods:

We used a holistic scheme combining whole-brain resting-state fMRI and graph theoretical analysis to examine the sustained effects on brain networks after administration of a single dose of ketamine and to identify the brain regions and circuits preferentially targeted by ketamine. Topological differences in functional networks of anaesthetised macaque monkeys were compared between ketamine (.5 mg/kg) and saline treatment after 18 hours.

Results:

We observed persistent global reconfiguration of small-world properties in response to ketamine intake, accompanied by large-scale down regulation of functional connectivity, most prominently in the orbital prefrontal cortex, the subgenual and posterior cingulate cortices, and the nucleus accumbens. Intriguingly, intrinsic connectivity with the medial prefrontal areas in the reward circuits were selectively down regulated. Global and regional regulations of the brain networks precisely opposed the maladaptive alterations in the depressed brain.

Conclusions:

Our results demonstrated that local synaptic plasticity triggered by blockade of N-methyl-D-aspartic acid receptors was capable of translating into prolonged network reconfiguration in the distributed cortico-limbic-striatal circuit, providing mechanistic insight into developing specific loci or circuit-targeted, long-term therapeutics.[9]

Similar findings have emerged from a randomised double-blind placebo-controlled trial in healthy human subjects with the observed changes occurring in 24 hours, matching the time course of the usual response to ketamine in treatment-resistant depressive conditions.[10]

Zanos et al in 2016 reported that the metabolism of ketamine was required before ketamine could work effectively in mice models of depression.[12] Specifically they found that 2R, 6R hydroxynorketamine [HNK] was the most potent metabolite in terms of antidepressant effect. They further reported that the action of HNK was not related to binding at the NMDA receptor, rather it seemed to be working through AMPA receptors. In addition HNK seemed to act without inducing some of the side effects that are seen with ketamine, in particular there was no indication of abuse potential.

Although there has been ongoing debate about these findings they have lead to further investigations into HNK as an antidepressant in its own right.

In humans delivering ketamine by the oral route gives greater proportions of HNK overall compared to the other routes of administration, potentially making this route a more effective strategy for the treatment of depression.

Moving on to a little known part of the brain. The human habenula is located next to the third ventricle above the thalamus, and is approximately 5-9 mm in diameter.

Human studies have noted that there are changes in electrical activity in this area in depressed patients and that deep brain stimulation involving the habenula can improve depressive symptoms.

Two new studies in rodents have explored the activity of this centre, which is thought to be involved in the processing of unexpectedly unpleasant events. It has been suggested that if the lateral habenula is overactive this could suppress the positive feelings that arise from usually pleasurable activities, this 'anhedonia' being a common symptom of depression.

Yan Yang et al noted a distinctive pattern of neuronal firing ["bursts"] in the lateral habenula of rats and mice displaying depression-like behaviours.[13] By inducing these bursts of activity by photostimulation they were able to produce depressive behaviours. They then infused ketamine directly into this area and found that the burst firing was rapidly reduced, as were the depressive behaviours – notably fluoxetine [Prozac] applied to the same area did not have this effect.

A second study by Cui et al examined the causes of the burst firing in depressed rats.[14] They found that a protein [Kir4.1] was present at higher levels in the astrocytes [see below] in the lateral habenula. These higher levels of Kir4.1 were associated with depressive behaviours and reducing these levels improved the behaviours.

Hence lifting the inhibition of the reward centres brought about by over activity of the lateral habenula is the suggested process for remission of rodent depression. The usual caveats of need for replication and the problems of translating from animals to human brains apply.

There have been further studies on astrocytes, which are star-shaped cells surrounding neurones in the brain and the spinal cord. Among their many functions they act to support repair processes in axons and synapses.

Lipid rafts:
It has been shown that conventional antidepressants act to move G-proteins off lipid rafts; storage areas found in in cell membranes. This movement then leads to increased neuronal activity.

Ketamine, in doses equivalent to human trials, has now been shown by Wray et al to move the G-proteins off the rafts more quickly than standard antidepressants i.e. in 15 minutes compared to 3 days.[15] The G –proteins also stay off the rafts for longer following ketamine administration.

One of the consequences of G-proteins becoming active is the increasing level of brain-derived neurotrophic factor [BDNF], this being seen from 24 hours after the ketamine infusion. BDNF is important for both dendrite growth and synapse formation.

Thus the researchers have demonstrated both an immediate and a delayed effect following ketamine application which appears to be independent of NMDA blockade and is also seen with the ketamine metabolite 2R, 6R hydroxynorketamine.

Ly et al. in their 2018 study showed that psychedelic compounds such as LSD increase neurogenesis and dendritic arbor complexity, promote dendritic spine growth, and stimulate synapse formation, thus promoting neuroplasticity.[16] These cellular effects are similar to those produced by ketamine and highlight the potential of psychedelics for treating depression and related disorders.

Another 2018 publication is this work from Williams et al exploring the role of opioid receptors in ketamine's therapeutic effect.[17] In a small cross-over study using intravenous ketamine in 12 patients with treatment-resistant depression, the authors found that giving the opioid antagonist naltrexone prior to injecting ketamine appeared to block the antidepressant effect, suggesting that a functioning opioid system is important for clinical improvement.

The study stopped early due to the clear-cut results.

The 12 patients were given 0.5mg/kg bodyweight of intravenous ketamine preceded either by 50mg of naltrexone or placebo.

Crossover occurred after 30 days.

7 of the 12 patients in the ketamine and placebo group responded in 24 hours post-infusion with the placebo and naltrexone group response being significantly lower.

There was no difference in dissociative symptoms between the two groups suggesting that achieving dissociation was not related to improvement.

Previous work using different doses of naltrexone has given different outcomes so this study does require replication.

One of the more-common observations by doctors about patients who have responded positively to ketamine has been their ability to make radical changes to their ways of viewing and acting in the world. This is in accord with the views of those who have combined ketamine with psychotherapy.

> 48 Year Old Female Psychologist 132 lbs. ketamine 25 mg. One Session. (This dose reflects a slight reduction from the research-based dose of 0.5 mg/kg due to the patient's request. It was given intramuscularly rather than through IV drip infusion.) Diagnosis: Bipolar Affective Disorder—Type I, depressed.
>
> The patient is a highly intelligent mental health professional with a convincing history of bipolar affective disorder. She had fallen into a depressive episode in the context of two concurrent stressors—ending a 7-year relationship and experiencing professional career difficulties that included a feeling of betrayal by a previous mentor. The patient usually performed effectively and efficiently at her work despite her deep vulnerability to questions of self-worth. Through previous therapeutic work she had developed the tools and strength needed to deal with a strongly critical sense of self, but these acute losses were proving to be too much this time.
>
> After six weeks her mood continued to deteriorate despite increasing her dose of valproic acid and other minor

changes in her medication regimen. Ketamine therapy was initiated and her Beck Depression Index dropped from 19 at treatment to three the next day. Two weeks later it had only risen to a score of seven, and two months later it was six. Her powerful response may be partially due to previously cultivated introspective skills and her capacity to make effective use of psychological insight. Her description of a rapid realignment and connection to deep internal resources characterised by love and forgiveness speaks for itself.

Following are her words in a voice message (permission given): 'I have been feeling amazing all week honestly. The depression is completely lifted. So, I'm on day seven and I still have zero depression. It really was a kind of truth serum for me. I've realised that those insights we discussed after the session are really all of the things that I already know about myself . . . but without all of the inhibitory thoughts in the way. It was about embracing myself and the love that I feel, which is at the core of my sense of meaning. It's just been an unbelievable week since that experience.'[11]

In summary, we can view a depressive illness as a disease of disconnection at a personal and social level and even more profoundly at the cellular level. Ketamine, through its action on the glutamate system, induces changes in both the quality and quantity of connections between neurons, and this in turn improves the function of critical brain circuits impaired by depression, thus freeing people to deal with their problems more effectively.

References

1. H. L. Mencken (paraphrased).
2. Janna Lawrence, 'The Secret Life of Ketamine', *The Pharmaceutical Journal* (March 2015).

2a Jon Hamilton 'Could a club drug offer almost immediate relief from depression?' http://www.npr.org/sections/health-shots/2012/01/30/145992588

3. N. Li, B. Lee, R. J. Liu, M. Banasr, J. M. Dwyer, M. Iwata, X. Y. Li, G. Aghajanian, R. S. Duman, 'mTOR-Dependent Synapse Formation Underlies the Rapid Antidepressant Effects of NMDA Antagonists', *Science*, 329/5994 (20 Aug 2010), 959–64. DOI: 10.1126/science.1190287.

4. O. H. Miller, L. Yang, C. C. Wang, E. A. Hargroder, Y. Zhang, E. Delpire, B. J. Hall, 'GluN2B-Containing NMDA Receptors Regulate Depression-Like Behavior and Are Critical for the Rapid Antidepressant Actions of Ketamine', *eLife*, 3 (2014), e03581. DOI: 10.7554/eLife.03581.

5. Nicolas D. Iadarola, Mark J. Niciu, Erica M. Richards, Jennifer L. Vande Voort, Elizabeth D. Ballard, Nancy B. Lundin, Allison C. Nugent, Rodrigo Machado-Vieira, and Carlos A. Zarate Jr, 'Ketamine and Other N-Methyl-D-Aspartate Receptor Antagonists in the Treatment of Depression: A Perspective Review', *Therapeutic Advances Chronic Diseases*. 2015 May; 6(3): 97–114. DOI: 10.1177/2040622315579059.

6. L. A. Opler, M. G. Opler, A. F. Arnsten, 'Ameliorating Treatment-Refractory Depression with Intranasal Ketamine: Potential NMDA Receptor Actions in the Pain Circuitry Representing Mental Anguish', *CNS Spectrums*, 26 (January 2015), 1–11.

7. Manabu Fuchikami, Alexandra Thomas, Rongjian Liu, Eric S. Wohleb, Benjamin B. Land, Ralph J. DiLeone, George K. Aghajanian, and Ronald S. Duman, 'Optogenetic Stimulation of Infralimbic PFC Reproduces Ketamine's Rapid and Sustained Antidepressant Actions', *Proceedings of the National Academy of Sciences*, 112/26, 8106–8111. DOI: 10.1073/pnas.1414728112.

8. R. H. Kaiser, J. R. Andrews-Hanna, T. D. Wager, D. A. Pizzagalli, 'Large-Scale Network Dysfunction in Major Depressive Disorder: A Meta-Analysis of Resting-State Functional Connectivity', *JAMA Psychiatry*, 72/6 (1 June 2015), 603–11. DOI: 10.1001/jamapsychiatry.2015.0071.

9. Qian Lva, Liqin Yanga, Guoliang Lib, Zhiwei Wanga, Zhuangming Shena, Wenwen Yua, Qinying Jianga, Baoyu Houa, Jian Pua, Hailan Hua, Zheng Wanga, 'Large-scale Persistent Network Reconfiguration Induced by Ketamine in Anesthetized Monkeys: Relevance to Mood Disorders', *Biological Psychiatry* (27 February 2015).

10. Milan Scheidegger, Martin Walter, Mick Lehmann, Coraline Metzger, Simone Grimm, Heinz Boeker, Peter Boesiger, Anke Henning, and Erich Seifritz, 'Ketamine Decreases Resting State Functional Network Connectivity in Healthy Subjects: Implications for Antidepressant Drug Action', *PLoS One*, 7/9 (24 September 2012), e44799. DOI: 10.1371/journal.pone.0044799.

11. Jeffrey Becker, 'Regarding the Transpersonal Nature of Ketamine Therapy: An Approach to the Work', *International Journal of Transpersonal Studies*, 33/2 (2014), 151–159.

New References:

12. Zanos, P., Moaddel, R., Morris, P. J., Georgiou, P., Fischell, J., Elmer, G. I., . . . Gould, T. D. (2016). NMDAR inhibition-independent antidepressant actions of ketamine metabolites. Nature, 533(7604), 481-486. doi: 10.1038/nature17998

13. Yang, Y., Cui, Y., Sang, K., Dong, Y., Ni, Z., Ma, S., & Hu, H. (2018). Ketamine blocks bursting in the lateral habenula to rapidly relieve depression. Nature, 554, 317. doi: 10.1038/nature25509

14. Cui, Y., Yang, Y., Ni, Z., Dong, Y., Cai, G., Foncelle, A., . . . Hu, H. (2018). Astroglial Kir4.1 in the lateral habenula drives neuronal bursts in depression. Nature, 554, 323. doi: 10.1038/nature25752

15. Wray, N. H., Schappi, J. M., Singh, H., Senese, N. B., & Rasenick, M. M. (2018). NMDAR-independent, cAMP-dependent antidepressant actions of ketamine. Molecular Psychiatry. doi: 10.1038/s41380-018-0083-8

16. Ly, C., Greb, A. C., Cameron, L. P., Wong, J. M., Barragan, E. V., Wilson, P. C., . . . Olson, D. E. (2018). Psychedelics Promote Structural and Functional Neural Plasticity. Cell Reports, 23(11), 3170-3182. doi: 10.1016/j.celrep.2018.05.022

17. Williams, N. R., Heifets, B. D., Blasey, C., Sudheimer, K., Pannu, J., Pankow, H., . . . Schatzberg, A. F. (2018). Attenuation of Antidepressant Effects of Ketamine by Opioid Receptor Antagonism. American Journal of Psychiatry, appi.ajp.2018.18020138. doi: 10.1176/appi.ajp.2018.18020138

Chapter 6

Is It Safe?

And so to medicine's first ethical principle: Do the potential benefits exceed the potential harm?

I have explored in previous chapters the positives of ketamine use in the treatment of depression; now for balance, let us examine the negatives.

Doctors have gained considerable knowledge about ketamine both through its use for anaesthesia over the past 50 years and in pain management for more than 20 years. In fact, ketamine is one of the most studied of all the medications available to us. Even with full anaesthesia, which uses doses up to ten times those prescribed for depression, ketamine is remarkably safe. A review of over 70,000 published anaesthesia cases reported only one ketamine-related fatality occurring and that in a seriously medically compromised individual.[1]

With the relatively low doses used to treat depression, the most common side effects are dry mouth, light-headedness, sleepiness, incoordination, dizziness, and nausea. Other less common experiences reported include feelings of unreality, euphoria, and anxiety as well as blurred vision, disorientation, and hallucinations. However, these symptoms have usually resolved an hour after the administration of ketamine.

Two factors that greatly influence the likelihood of experiencing side effects are the dose and the route of administration. The speed of absorption of ketamine into the body is fastest by the intravenous route and slowest for the oral for an equivalent dose, and the frequency and severity of reported side effects seem to correlate directly to this. Another important influence is the setting in which the treatment takes place; a calm environment and positive support from trusted therapists are associated with more positive experiences. It is noteworthy that the two studies showing the lowest positive responses to IV ketamine for depression were conducted in busy hospital areas.

The short-term side effects from ketamine treatment noted in studies over the past 15 years are detailed in the comprehensive review by Ryan et al. in 2014, who summarised the adverse effects of ketamine treatment reported from 79 trials involving 550 patients.[2]

They noted that for those receiving IV ketamine, there were just two problems during the infusion process which led to cessation of treatment; the first was related to low blood pressure, and the second involved high blood pressure that was unresponsive to antihypertensives at the time. After the infusion, four patients ceased treatment due to worsening depressive symptoms and anxiety. Two placebo patients also discontinued—one due to anxiety and one because of elevated blood pressure.

In case reports, one patient receiving S-ketamine discontinued during infusion due to dissociation, which is interesting as S-ketamine has been thought to be less likely to induce dissociative side effects.

Increased heart rate and transient increases in blood pressure were commonly noted haemodynamic effects in the trials. There was one report of a patient with slowed breathing and a temporary reduction in oxygen levels during a ketamine infusion. No trials have reported any haemodynamic effects persisting beyond 4 hours save for one patient with mild, asymptomatic low blood pressure, which persisted for 24 hours.

Dissociation, psychotomimetic effects, manic symptoms, and other psychiatric effects were measured in most studies. These side effects were measured by a variety of rating scales and revealed significant increases compared with baseline levels that generally resolved within four hours.

In the four studies using repeated dosing, changes in psychiatric and physical symptoms were similar after each infusion, with no progressive increase with multiple infusions. Increased doses of ketamine were associated with increases in dissociative symptoms in one ascending-dose study in which IV infusions over two to five minutes, an unusually rapid administration, were used.

One suicide attempt occurred during the washout period prior to ketamine treatment. One report of mania was noted in a patient who received 34 doses of ketamine at variable intervals over a 1-year period. Another study reported a 'mild' hypomanic episode in a patient after his third infusion. There have been reports of short-term euphoria during the treatment process.

Reports of side effects from case studies have been consistent with the more formal trials, and notably there have been no unusual side effects noted with repeated administration of ketamine over periods of up to two years.

Ryan also examined the different administration routes, noting that for intramuscular ketamine, the adverse effects were very similar to intravenous use. One report indicated a decrease of dissociative symptoms following repeated injections.

From the Papolos study of intranasal ketamine for paediatric patients, brief dissociative effects similar to the IV route were reported as well as mild palpitations and, for one patient, moderate respiratory distress. In a second intranasal case report, the patient described feeling high during the first few of more than 30 administrations.

From Lara's study of low-dose sublingual ketamine in 26 patients, there were no reported euphoric, psychotic, or dissociative symptoms. Transient light-headedness and, in one report, increased heart rate for less than 30 minutes occurred. Mouth numbness was the only novel effect reported.

For oral ketamine, the 50 patients experienced few adverse effects save for disorientation and hallucinations in a minority of a medically ill hospice population. In fact, for many, there were improvements in adverse-symptom checklists. Only diarrhoea, trouble sleeping, and trouble sitting still occurred (one each) in a study of 14 patients. One study of oral S-ketamine taken three times daily found essentially no side effects in all four patients.

In addition, follow-ups of both healthy subjects and patients with psychotic illnesses who were given ketamine in the 1990s did not reveal any problems related to their taking the drug; specifically, there were no reports of drug abuse or psychosis.

Diligent monitoring in clinic or hospital settings is essential for ketamine injection treatment as well as for higher-dose oral, sublingual, and intranasal delivery.

However, learning from the experience of our colleagues in pain medicine, it appears that low-dose oral and sublingual ketamine after an initial monitored test dose can be safely continued in the home setting.[3]

As to the long-term side effects, we again can profit from the experiences of pain clinicians who have used both daily long-term sublingual ketamine and repeated, continuous (for five to ten days) intravenous infusions to treat severe chronic pain conditions.

From them, we have learned the following:

1. Serial, continuous intravenous infusions can rarely cause raised liver enzymes, which return to normal levels on discontinuation of the ketamine. No elevation of liver enzymes has been reported from the use of single infusions.

2. These infusions also can occasionally cause bladder symptoms, which again are short-lived.

3. There are no reports from patients treated with these infusions of long-term problems with concentration or memory, nor is there evidence of abuse or addiction occurring despite some having multiple treatments over many years.

4. Sublingual ketamine given daily for up to 18 years for pain conditions has not been associated with worrying side effects, nor have there been reports indicating tolerance, dependence, or addiction in this group.

As to fears that patients who have been given take-home doses of ketamine may use it to overdose, 'it is a drug of abuse at high dosages, but very safe and effective when given under direct medical supervision. How safe and how high? The lethal dose of Ketamine is estimated to be 450 times the typical dose given for depression. Water is lethal at a dozen 16-ounce glasses of water in one sitting. Yes, in many ways Ketamine is as safe as water, when handled properly.'[4]

Abuse and Addiction—the Dark Side

There is no doubt that regular long-term recreational use of ketamine can lead to tolerance (the need to increase doses to get the desired effect), dependence, and addiction in 5–10% of this group. As well as potential addiction, there are a range of hazards that ketamine recreational users face, beginning with the doubt as to whether they are getting what they have paid for. Some are unaware of the possible consequences of their usage, and many are confirmed risk-takers.

'With street ketamine, there's no way to know what ingredients you're putting into the batter. One small study tested several dozen samples of club drugs, including ketamine, bought illegally on the New York club scene. It found that 100% of them were adulterated with other substances, ranging from Epsom salt to cocaine. Some supposed ketamine samples contained *zero* Ketamine. In some cases the buyers were certain they got pure, genuine ketamine because it came in the manufacturer's packaging (a vial of liquid solution). But even those were adulterated. Much of the ketamine solution had been removed with a syringe and non-sterile fluid was injected back into the vial so it appeared full, which diluted the strength of what remained and also introduced microorganisms.'[5]

Karl Jansen, whose book *Ketamine: Dreams and Realities* is a gold mine of information on the early days of ketamine, also had this to say:[6] 'When ketamine is used in uncontrolled settings recreationally, it can lead to significant medical problems, including excessive sedation and respiratory depression especially if combined with depressants like alcohol, benzodiazepines, or gamma hydroxybutyrate [GHB or fantasy].'

As to the physical risks, he added, 'In non-medical use the real physical dangers arise mainly from the setting, as ketamine can leave the taker in a helpless and/or confused state. Difficulty with balance, combined with numbness, muscle weakness and impaired vision, has resulted in falls which were sometimes lethal. The analgesia has resulted in severe burns, and lying down has resulted in ulnar nerve compression in the arm where the body was lying on it. Other risks from the setting are drowning, death by hypothermia from lying outside in winter, traffic accidents and becoming a crime victim (e.g. 'sedate rape'). D. M. Turner died in 1997, aged 34, having drowned in a bathtub with a bottle of ketamine at his side. He appears to have collapsed into the water, after ignoring his own harm minimisation advice about not injecting alone while engaged in activities such as bathing. This accidental death illustrates the dangers of becoming helpless in settings other than lying down on a bed. Some of the physical effects of principal concern in a non-medical use context are difficulty with walking and balance resulting in falls, numbness, slurred or hoarse speech, dizziness, visual problems, vertigo, nausea and vomiting, headaches, sweating, muscle spasms, and twitches, sudden jerky movements and tremor.'

Those who commonly combine ketamine with other illegal substances and alcohol and whose lifestyle and self-care are not optimal are at risk of serious harm. There have now been over 200 patients reported as having ketamine-related bladder problems, causing considerable pain and distress. In some, the damage has been sufficiently severe that their bladders have had to be removed.

To put this in context, ketamine addicts often take more than 3 g of ketamine daily—100 times the typical starting dose for intravenous ketamine for depression. One Spanish study by Garcia Larrosa of 14 long-term recreational-ketamine users stated: 'Six patients (46%) reported LUTS [bladder symptoms] with daily mean micturitions every 42 minutes and night-time of 3 episodes, with dysuria (100%), urgency (100%), incontinence (20%), decreased flow (80%), hypogastric or perineal pain (80%), gross haematuria (80%) and bilateral lumbar spine pain (40%). Symptomatic patients described a mean intake of inhaled ketamine of 3 g/day, 80% taking the drug daily and the asymptomatic ones of 1.03 g/day limited to weekends. The mean consumption time to the appearance of the symptoms was 31 months. Intensity of the symptoms was related to the ketamine dose and improved on increasing water intake.'[7]

Other reported problems of regular high-dose ketamine use include abdominal pain, liver and bile duct damage, memory problems, and paranoid thinking.

According to Jansen again:

> Many agencies now have leaflets about 'Special K,' some of which are more accurate than others. The commonest mistakes in these leaflets are claims that ketamine is a 'downer,' as it is more likely to act as a stimulant, to focus on 'overdose' (usually not an issue) and vomiting (not as common

as often claimed, unless the user has been drinking), and not to mention that the main danger is falling over. However, high frequency users can become over-confident and very full of themselves, and may have a tendency to ignore any advice on the basis that they know far more about everything, and ketamine in particular, than other people do. They feel that they are a special case. They may even feel inclined to give advice to others from which they themselves may be excused, as in the cases of D. M. Turner and John Lilly [early ketamine psychonauts or mind explorers]. Advice given to them is often ignored, especially after the first dose takes effect. Nevertheless, some basic harm minimisation advice will be stated here, in the hope that some good may come of it.

The only way to have no direct risk from a drug is not to take it. There is still indirect risk, such as being injured by a drunken driver. Once the decision has been made to proceed, the next step in reducing risk is to take the smallest dose required to provide the desired effect, by the safest route in the safest possible setting route.

One of the biggest risks we face, due to the very slow progress in bringing ketamine treatment to patients, is that people will literally take the matter into their own hands and seek illegal supplies in order to self-medicate. This is not recommended as the product is often not true to description and the consequences of misuse can be severe. In online forums, people regularly talk of getting carried away and using far more ketamine than they had planned.

It is also important to know that when considering the potential for abuse and addiction in the 50 years since ketamine began to be given to humans for medical reasons, reports that this has led to abuse, dependence, or addiction are very rare. One guesstimate is that less than one in two hundred patients could potentially be affected. This does not mean that abuse cannot or will not occur, nor should we be reckless in our prescribing, but it does indicate that the oft-repeated fears expressed by some researchers are exaggerated.

Carlos Zarate, one of the most experienced researchers of ketamine for depression, has commented, 'For the most part, ketamine is well tolerated, with mild to moderate side effects. When you ask patients, they say the pain of experiencing depression is much more than five or ten minutes of these dissociative effects. And a lot of these patients have been on other medications for decades and have experienced the side effects of these drugs, so it has to be put in the context of that too.'

Dennis Charney, co-author of the original Yale study and dean of Icahn School of Medicine at Mount Sinai stated, 'We give chemotherapy for cancer and there are side effects with chemotherapy, but we give it anyway, because people need it to get better from cancer. Ketamine does not have the side effects chemotherapy does, yet we're using it for a disease that has a defined mortality; there is a suicide rate associated with severe depression.'

And Dennis Hartman from the Ketamine Advocacy Network had this to say, 'There is a philosophical question as to whether depression in any severity justifies the potential risk of indefinite use of ketamine? Well, the question has been answered in the affirmative, with little debate, for other illnesses and ketamine. Sufferers of Complex Regional Pain Syndrome receive multiple, extremely high dose ketamine for the rest of their lives. Major burn survivors would probably have the lifetime load of 100 ketamine patients. As a survivor of bipolar depression, my vote is clearly on the side of balanced risk and reward.'

For all the focus on peer-reviewed published work it is important to remember that many patients and clinicians have not been content to wait until all researchers have fully satisfied their doubts as to the balance of long term benefits and harms with ketamine therapy, but instead have cautiously gone ahead with treatment, embracing the uncertainty. Most of the published studies to date have come from academic institutions, but there is now extensive reported evidence from doctors around the world who have been treating "real" patients, i.e. those with comorbidities and those who are suicidal.

For psychiatric disorders in the USA, Drs. Brooks Levine and Mandel have given accounts of more than 3,500 patients they have treated over the years without serious side effects including dependence and addiction.

Dr. Glen Brooks, a 67-year-old anaesthesiologist, opened New York Ketamine Infusions in 2012 following a family tragedy.[8] Over the past six years Dr. Brooks has administered ketamine to more than 2,000 patients in his Manhattan office.

Dr. Steven Levine is the founder of Actify Neurotherapies, a group which has given over 1800 patients more than 20,000 ketamine infusions and now operates from 10 locations.[9] He strongly advocates for treatment protocols and registries and is the vice-president of the American Society of Ketamine Physicians [ASKP].

Dr. Steve Mandel, the current President of the ASKP, has treated more than 600 patients to date, indicating that he has administered more than 4,000 ketamine infusions, and he has reported an 83% effectiveness rate—higher than the reported rate in the literature and research at large of around 70 percent. [10] His youngest patient to date has been 15, and his oldest 88.

Angelo De Gioannis [see chapters 3 and 7] and colleagues have now treated over 800 patients over the past 5 years using oral ketamine in their community clinic in Brisbane, Australia.[11]

Their overall response and remission rates are similar to those obtained by practitioners using ketamine by injection. In addition they have noted low rates of problematic side effects and in a recent study found many of their patients on maintenance oral ketamine reduced their dose over time.

In other domains e.g. pain management, many more patients have been prescribed ketamine, increasingly so since 2000.

With regards to the long-term safety of ketamine therapy there is a growing body of evidence particularly from pain physicians such as Varun Jaitly and Lucinda Grande.

Jaitly [see Chapter 7] has been treating patients with sublingual ketamine over the past eighteen years and has patients who have been taking daily doses for that time without significant problems, while Grande has described her experiences with more than 390 patients treated with oral and sublingual ketamine over the past five years with a very low rate of serious treatment complications.[12] Average doses for pain relief were 100mg.

As she observed:

"Addiction: Some find the use of higher doses to be pleasurable. Two of my patients sought to continually escalate the dose to the point where I wondered if the therapeutic effect had become secondary to the pleasurable experience. These two patients, whose behaviour might be described as addictive, represent 0.5% of the patients to whom I have initiated ketamine treatment.

Bladder pain: Three patients with pre-existing interstitial cystitis had to discontinue use of ketamine after a few weeks due to worsening of bladder pain. This is noteworthy because a study of long-term ketamine abusers found bladder ulceration in some."

Not all is rosy however...

Here is a very good example of how not to treat patients with ketamine.[13]

A man with a history of alcohol misuse and recurrent episodes of depression with suicide attempts obtained a supply of ketamine in large amounts on a monthly basis from an interstate provider without ongoing face to face contact or adequate monitoring. The prescribed daily doses of up to 900mg daily taken intranasally were extremely high and the patient at times reported taking twice that amount, obtaining relief from his depressive symptoms for only 2-3 hours. Several months after his prescriptions were stopped he died in a single car accident that the family considered was suicide – alcohol but not ketamine was found in his post-mortem blood test results.

In better news Dr. Jennifer Southgate in a presentation at the Oxford Ketamine conference in 2018 detailed the results of a prospective study of 183 patients exploring ketamine's potential effects on the bladder.[14]

9 of the 183 had elevated scores on a cystitis scale. However, all elevations were registered prior to ketamine's initiation.1 possible ketamine-related effect was noted with low initial score on the cystitis scale but increasing scores over 3 infusions.

Feifel et al from La Jolla, California also presented at the Oxford Ketamine conference on the results of a survey of physicians who are currently treating patients with parenteral [by injection] ketamine.[15]

They surveyed 99 known established providers of parenteral ketamine for depression - [there are now an estimated 1,000 providers and more than 250 "ketamine clinics" in the USA alone.]

49 providers responded of whom 60% were psychiatrists. In total they had treated a total of 7544 patients, 30% of whom had received

more than 10 infusions. 90% of the physicians considered ketamine to be as safe as, or safer than standard antidepressants.

81 patients [1%] had treatment discontinued due to adverse effects. [I'm aware that online comments suggest that the main reason patients cease treatment is the cost – typically up to $3000 for a course of 6 infusions].

The adverse effects included:

11 reports of bladder dysfunction [0.15%]
13 reports of possible addiction [.13%]
3 reports of psychosis [.04%]
2 reports of cognitive decline [.03%]

They concluded that these results suggest a very low rate of serious side effects. Taken together with the outcomes of Janssen's esketamine trials and reports from physicians who have been treating patients for many years now, we can be confident that the potential benefits of ketamine therapy far outweigh the known risks.

So both the short-term and the long-term side effects of ketamine treatment are predictable and manageable. Who then should consider trying ketamine, and who should not?

References

1. R. J. Strayer, L. S. Nelson, 'Adverse Events Associated with Ketamine for Procedural Sedation in Adults', *American Journal of Emergency Medicine*, 26/9 (November 2008), 985–1028. DOI: 10.1016/j.ajem.2007.12.005.

2. Wesley C. Ryan, 'Ketamine and Depression: A Review', *International Journal of Transpersonal Studies*, 33/2 (2014), 40–74.

3. V. K. Jaitly, 'Sublingual Ketamine in Chronic Pain: Service Evaluation by Examining More Than 200 Patient Years of Data', *Journal of Observational Pain Medicine*, 1/2 (2013).

4. Ketamine Advocacy Network.

5. Ibid.
6. Karl L. R. Jansen, *Ketamine: Dreams and Realities* (2001). Published by MAPS [Multidisciplinary Association for Psychedelic Studies] www.maps.org
7. Alejandro García-Larrosa, 'Urinary Tract Lesions Associated to Ketamine Consumption', *Medicina Clínica*, 143/8 (21/10/2014). DOI: 10.1016/j.medcli.2013.11.019.
8. "How ketamine went from dance floor drug to wonder pill." Arts +Culture News "From after party to doctor's surgery: we speak to a New York doctor who prescribes ketamine for depression and PTSD."
   Text Thomas Gorton
9. Levine Steven: DAILY NEWS CONTRIBUTOR Interview Friday, September 1, 2017, 5:10 PM.
10. Mandel Steve. "Ketamine Could Be the New Depression Treatment of Choice. The strange journey of the party drug that may be the key to rewiring the brain." Tierney Finster MEL Magazine, Oct 2017.
11. Grande Lucinda MD "Sublingual Ketamine for Chronic Pain and/or Depression. Information for Prescribers. 28/12/2017 Personal communication, available on request.
12. Hartberg, J., Garrett-Walcott, S., & De Gioannis, A. (2018). Impact of oral ketamine augmentation on hospital admissions in treatment-resistant depression and PTSD: a retrospective study. Psychopharmacology, 235(2), 393-398. doi: 10.1007/s00213-017-4786-3
13. Schak, K. M., Vande Voort, J. L., Johnson, E. K., Kung, S., Leung, J. G., Rasmussen, K. G., . . . Frye, M. A. (2016). Potential Risks of Poorly Monitored Ketamine Use in Depression Treatment. American Journal of Psychiatry, 173(3), 215-218. doi: 10.1176/appi.ajp.2015.15081082
14. Southgate et al. Oxford Conference abstract 2018.
15. Feifel et al "Safety of Treating Depression with ketamine in the real world." Oxford conference abstract 2018.

Chapter 7

The Ketamine Doctors

Introduction

During the time I have been researching and treating patients with ketamine, I have been able to make contact with a number of pioneers in the field. Each became involved with ketamine for different reasons, but what they have in common is the awareness that our current therapies are often ineffective and that we must be open to new opportunities. Trailblazers in any endeavour need energy and passion; they must overcome many hurdles. And it's all too easy to become discouraged not least through the indifference, disbelief, and at times, outright opposition from their peers.

I have been struck by the extraordinary generosity shown to me by these doctors who have so willingly shared their knowledge and experience. Unfortunately, there will always be some in any endeavour whose chief motivation is fame or fortune, but these doctors are driven by a more important desire—to do more to help people who are suffering.

There are other practitioners, chiefly working in the United States, who have gained much experience in working with ketamine. In particular I would like to acknowledge Drs. Glen Brooks, Steven Levine, Lucinda Grande, Steve Mandel, Paul Glue, Phil Wolfson and Ian McShane, who are mentioned elsewhere in this book. I would encourage readers to visit their websites and learn more about their ideas and methods as the world of ketamine is wide and there are many different treatment approaches that are proving to be helpful.

So here's a selection of ketamine doctors: Angelo De Gioannis, whose incredible work has to date largely flown under the radar; Graham Barrett, who had more exposure than he wished for; Diogo Lara, whose study of sublingual ketamine inspired my efforts with this approach; and Varun Jaitly, whose practical and consistent approach to using sublingual ketamine for pain conditions over the past 18 years has given all more confidence concerning the safety of prescribing low-dose ketamine for extended periods.

Angelo De Gioannis

When Angelo De Gioannis was contemplating moving from Rome to Australia in 1999, he was told in no uncertain terms by his wife that they had to 'go somewhere warm'. This proved to be Brisbane's gain and Tasmania's loss, but what it did give him was access to a large pool of patients with treatment-resistant depression.

An early interest in the assessment and management of suicidal patients led him to join the staff of the Australian Institute for Suicide Research and Prevention at the Griffith University, where he is now a senior lecturer. There he published with co-author Diego De Leo the article 'Managing Suicidal Patients in Clinical Practice' in 2012.[1]

In 2014 Angelo and Diego wrote a letter to the *Australian Journal of Psychiatry* on the treatment of two patients with suicidal thoughts and depression using oral ketamine.[2]

To the Editor:

In a recent article in this journal the effectiveness of intravenous Ketamine in treatment resistant depression was highlighted. The following case reports describe the use of oral ketamine as augmentation treatment in patients presenting with chronic suicide ideation and at least two significant past suicide attempts.

Mr. B was a 44 year old man with a history of bipolar depression and chronic suicide ideation since adolescence. His condition was further complicated by severe chronic pain and a family history of suicide. Despite multiple pharmacotherapy combinations, and the current regime of amitryptiline (200 mg nocte) and quetiapine (100 mg b.i.d.), he remained depressed, with scores of 36 on the MADRS and 4/6 on the suicide item. Following written informed consent, oral ketamine was added. The treatment involved fortnightly doses of a ketamine solution (100 mg/ml) ingested orally with a flavoured drink. Starting with an initial dose of 0.5 mg/kg and gradually increasing by 0.5 mg/kg with each treatment, we achieved sustained clinical response at around 3 mg/kg without any adverse or side effects. Within 24 hours of his first treatment his score on MADRS and suicide item decreased to 17 and 1, respectively. Repeated treatments every two to three weeks produced sustained remission of his suicidal ideation.

Mrs. A was a 37 year old woman with bipolar depression and suicide ideation since adolescence. Her medication history included adequate trials of venlafaxine, mirtazapine, fluoxetine, quetiapine, olanzapine and several courses of ECT. Her current regime included venlafaxine (150 mg q.d.) and quetiapine (700 mg q.d.). She remained depressed with scores on MADRS and suicidality of 31 and 4 respectively. After obtaining written informed consent, oral ketamine was added. The initial dose of 0.5 mg/kg was gradually increased to 1.5 mg/kg. Within 24 hours from her first treatment the scores decreased to 10 on the MADRS and 2 on the suicide item. She continued to receive monthly doses of oral ketamine and her mental state continued to improve with no suicide ideation between treatments.

Pre-treatment blood tests included liver function tests and CBC with differential. Blood pressure and pulse rate were monitored before and 30 minutes after each dose. Neither patient experienced adverse events or significant changes in vital signs during the treatment.

Although case reports require cautious consideration, these results are consistent with recent findings supporting the use of ketamine in treating severe depression. The possibility of using oral ketamine as a viable alternative to IV ketamine infusion is of special interest.

Angelo first became interested in ketamine when a patient's father, who was an anaesthetist, suggested he try it for his son who was severely depressed and suicidal.

Ultimately, Angelo did not prescribe ketamine as his patient improved before he could get the treatment organised, but he began reading more and more about it.

Before starting to treat patients with ketamine, he had discussions with various state and federal government authorities as well as with the local Drugs of Dependence Unit. His aim was 'not to set up an empire' but to explore the viability of using oral and sublingual ketamine in a clinic setting.

He, with colleague Johann Scheepers, then established a clinic where they explored the use of initially sublingual and then oral ketamine in combination with emotion modulation therapy (EMT). EMT is a mode of psychotherapy developed at the Australian Institute for Suicide Research and Prevention. It helps patients to improve their ability to cope with problems in life and reduce the level of discomfort in approaching everyday challenges. EMT has been used to treat a wide range of disorders, including depression, anxiety, and personality disorders.

Now six years later, Angelo has treated more than 800 patients, with an estimated overall 75% response rate and a 50% remission rate. Angelo sees ketamine as a way of unlocking potential and freeing up patients to change from maladaptive coping strategies to healthier approaches, thereby reducing the risk of relapse in the longer term. Overall, Angelo believes that ketamine is a very helpful aid but very much a part of a larger picture.

The treatment process begins with an initial assessment following referral and a physical review by a general practitioner. Importantly, all patients must be in active psychotherapy with Angelo or other therapists. After information about the treatment is discussed and consent forms signed, patients take a starting dose of 0.3–0.5 mg/kg body weight, which is split into in two separate doses.

He monitors the response, checking both blood pressure and pulse rates, and aims for the feeling of mild inebriation similar to that felt after having a glass of wine to establish whether a sufficient brain level of ketamine has been reached. He titrates the dose over the next two to four weeks, giving two doses a day twice weekly when possible.

After a typical starting oral dose of 40 mg, given mixed with fruit juice to mask the bitterness, he builds to an average dose of 200 mg daily and as much as 600 mg if necessary.

He reasons that giving two doses in the day three hours apart will allow a larger amount to be taken without excessive side effects, this being a method used for people being treated with ketamine for chronic pain. Taking higher doses in a day, he also thought, will help the patient to reach an effective dose more quickly.

In most cases, patients take two doses of ketamine in a day and attend EMT-focused consultations initially to assess progress (partners are often involved) and to help patients to identify triggers for mood changes, to recognise their bodily reactions to stressors, and to develop a range of strategies for managing these situations, including the use of p.r.n. (taken episodically when needed) medication.

Angelo has found that tolerance to the side effects of ketamine does not always occur. If anything, once a maximum dose has been reached, this dose needs to be lowered as patients seem to become more sensitive to the unwanted effects as they improve. He initially continues a patient's usual medications but finds over time that these doses also need to be reduced due to the increased levels of side effects.

He has observed increases in blood pressure and pulse rates in the hour after ketamine administration, but no one has required active intervention. Also, some patients develop dissociative symptoms and hallucinations, which disappear over time with reassurance and the occasional use of diazepam. Interestingly in this regard, research by anaesthetists has established that positive suggestions given prior to giving ketamine have positive effects on the experience, allowing it to be more interesting and enjoyable.[3]

Angelo began by treating patients with the sublingual route of administration but concluded after a few months that the oral route was simpler and also gave higher levels of norketamine and hydroxynorketamine. These are breakdown metabolites of ketamine and active in their own right. He has seen a few patients who have not responded to intravenous ketamine but have gone on to do well with the oral route.

The people who have responded best have been the younger patients with 'pure' depression (i.e. not complicated by personality disorders) or having gains such as financial benefits related to their illnesses. Those that have had fewer episodes of depression prior to treatment with ketamine often have a faster and more sustained response than those with the more chronic conditions. If a patient has not responded to six weeks of high doses of ketamine, Angelo will then discuss the other options available to them.

In 2018, as described in Chapter 3, Angelo and colleagues published the results of a retrospective study on the impact of oral ketamine on hospital admissions for patients with treatment-resistant depression and PTSD.

Angelo concludes, 'I have no doubt that Ketamine works, the main issue is how to properly and safely manage the process of treatment.'

Graham Barrett

Associate Professor Graham Barrett is the head of laboratory at the University of Melbourne's Department of Physiology. He is a neuroscientist with a strong interest in neural plasticity and neurotropins and has widely published on these topics.

An active clinician, he has had 30 years' experience in treating depression.

In 2014 he became a consulting doctor for Aura Medical Services, a company set up to provide ketamine injections for patients with treatment-resistant depression. Aura then operated clinics in Melbourne, Sydney, and Brisbane. The treatment program involved the administration of 40–60 mg of ketamine subcutaneously (by injection under the skin) twice a week for six weeks (at $150 per injection), then one injection a week for another six weeks. However, doses and treatment duration varied dramatically, with some patients spending up to $3,000 on a course of treatment. Aura by early 2015 had treated 'over 500 patients with a 65% success rate for patients with severe depression'.

Graham personally had treated 50 patients, with 90% having severe treatment-resistant depression non-responsive to multiple medications and, for some, to ECT. In these patients, the response rate had been 70–75%. Some patients had not required any further ketamine therapy while others continue to be treated, usually monthly. There had been no significant problems with side effects.

He had stated: 'If you take a hundred people with severe depression, 60 are adequately covered by antidepressants. That leaves 40 who aren't. If ketamine can relieve the suffering of 30 of those 40, that's a huge amount of suffering that's being relieved, that's a huge number of people who are getting their lives back.'

He believed that despite the drug's experimental status, it should be available to the public.

I do respect the opinion of the cautious types who say that it's premature. We don't know enough about it to let everyone start prescribing it; we've got to proceed with care. But it's safe, and it fills a need, and therefore it can be justified to use off-label. And by the way, if you took off-label prescribing out of medicine, doctors would be out of business. Off-label use of medications is much more common and frequent than is commonly realised.

There have now been over 30 studies in the US, and they're unanimous that ketamine works in 70 per cent of cases of resistant depression. Well, thirty studies are good enough for me.

The fact that ketamine is an older drug and its patent has long expired means that there's nothing in it for the drug companies. No drug company is going to pick up the tab of going through the extremely expensive process of running the clinical trials that you need in order for the drug to become registered by the TGA. That's an extremely expensive process and you've got to have a pot of gold at the end to induce a drug company to take it on. With ketamine there's no pot of gold.

So it's up to a small number of doctors who are either crusaders or entrepreneurs or a combination of both, who open ketamine clinics and make it available to people.

We've got a lot of hard research to be done, but I want to find out with ketamine how best to use it. How long does it work for? Do people come resistant to it? Can you give it for long periods of time? Do people develop a dependence on it? These are the questions that are interesting to me.

The US have done a lot more work there, way in advance of us. The number of studies done is now quite large, and so far there hasn't been any significant negative finding. I think that somehow or other we have allowed this party drug stigma to frighten us too much.

Patients who have been suffering for twenty-five years and have tried every antidepressant in the handbook, receive ketamine and get their old life back . . . their feeling of gratitude and happiness is overwhelming. They say, 'why haven't we been using this before?' The Americans are doing it, why haven't we been doing it? And it does come back to the stigma of being associated with a party drug.

Aura subsequently appeared in the news because of its association with another company, which had been the subject of legal proceedings. Graham then resigned from his position with Aura, having become increasingly concerned that Aura's focus on profits was beginning to diminish the standard of care his patients required. He no longer prescribes ketamine.

In an interview conducted by Tracy Bowden in 2015, Les, one of the patients Graham has treated explained,[3] 'Look, I was actually going really bad, scraping the bottom of the barrel and when you think about taking your own life, you've got to be really down to—in a pretty desperate sense of mind to even think about that.'

Tracy commented, 'He had tried several different antidepressant medications and underwent counselling, but nothing helped—until now. Today he's receiving the latest in a series of injections of a drug called ketamine.'

Les stated, 'I'm just so much better than what I was before. I can't put it into words really; it's that's good. I've, you know, gone back to some of my old interests, playing a bit of music and things like that, and actually getting—trying to get back to work and organise a business for myself. And it's good to actually find something that can battle the problem that you've been having after you've tried so many different avenues and then you get a successful one. It's been so good. It's really wonderful, it is.'

Diogo Lara

Diogo Lara, after training at the Universidade Federal do Rio Grande do Sul, completed his psychiatry degree and a PhD in biochemistry in 2000. He is now a full professor at the Pontificia Universidade

Católica do Rio Grande do Sul and a researcher at Conselho Nacional de Pesquisa, a national agency for research. He has had 128 articles published in PubMed indexed journals on psychiatry, behaviour, and psychopharmacology.

He explained when his interest in ketamine arose. 'I usually read the main journals in psychiatry and I was impressed with the first results. It was pretty obvious that other routes were possible, and I was starting with oral ketamine (only 2 patients), when I came across Dr Luciano Munari, a very smart psychiatrist who had been treating patients with very low dose ketamine since 2008. He gave me all the tips and I just started using it. Then we collected some cases and published our paper together.'

Thus, Diogo and his colleagues in Brazil in 2013 published the results of their trial of very-low-dose sublingual ketamine (VLDS) for the treatment of treatment-resistant unipolar and bipolar depression.[4] They had observed the published positive results from the series of trials using intravenous ketamine for depression.

They stated:

> Despite this conceptual advance, the need to submit patients to i.v. administration within a hospital setting is a strong limitation for a more widespread and continuous administration of ketamine. Thus, the application and maintenance of ketamine treatment depends on finding better routes of administration than i.v. Intramuscular injection at 1 mg/kg was efficacious in five case reports but is far from ideal. Ketamine after oral administration undergoes rapid first pass metabolism, resulting in only 17% bioavailability and high conversion to the metabolite norketamine, but there are three case reports of successful treatment with 0.5 mg/kg oral ketamine in patients receiving hospice care and two with refractory depression. Another alternative undergoing clinical trials is the use of a nasal spray, which renders a bioavailability of 45%. However, ketamine in the usual liquid form is not friendly to use intranasally and may produce erratic absorption. Surprisingly, the sublingual administration of ketamine has not been explored

but it renders 30% bioavailability and less conversion to norketamine than oral administration. This route can be easily used with liquid ketamine and allows providing a small amount (1 ml) to the patient in a dropper bottle to facilitate personal use while guaranteeing that the patient does not have access to a dose that can lead to anaesthesia or psychosis. Moreover, sublingual administration of drugs has been increasingly used for psychiatric drugs and is usually well accepted by patients.

Another issue that has been poorly studied is the dose-response curve for the antidepressant effects of ketamine. Since the original Berman study used an i.v. infusion of 0.5 mg/kg ketamine over 40 minutes, most studies since have just repeated the same protocol, but this dose selection was based on a serendipitous observation in a challenge study in depressed patients. Although this is considered a sub psychotomimetic dose, perceptual disturbances, drowsiness, euphoria, feeling 'strange', confusion and dissociation often occur at this dose. The reported efficacy of 0.5 mg/kg oral ketamine, which would lead to a bioavailability of 6 mg in a 70 kg subject, suggests that the habitual i.v. dose of 0.5 mg/kg (bioavailability of 30–35 mg in a 70 kg subject) is more than is actually necessary.

With these considerations in mind, we started evaluating the effects and tolerability of very low-dose, sublingual ketamine administered in outpatients with unipolar or bipolar refractory depressive episodes.

Diogo's team recruited 26 patients with severe treatment-resistant conditions and began treatment.

Method:

This study was conducted as an unsystematic case series in a clinical setting in patients who were explained the procedures and provided written informed consent. Patients included in this case series had to fulfil the DSM-IV criteria for major depression (single episode or recurrent) or bipolar disorder experiencing a depressive episode. They had to have unsatisfactory response to at least four pharmacological treatments indicated for their disorder, alone or in combination, for at least 4 weeks at standard therapeutic doses.

Our strategy was to start with a very low dose (0.1 ml=2 drops) of racemic ketamine 100 mg/ml (i.e. 10 mg) administered sublingually, allowed to absorb for 5 min and then swallowed. We then observed for acute therapeutic effects and increased the dose by 1 drop as needed in further doses on another day. Estimating the 30% bioavailability for this route, only 3 mg ketamine would be actually delivered at this starting dose, which is about 10 times lower than 35 mg in a 70 kg subject undergoing the classical i.v. administration of 0.5 mg/kg (93% bioavailability) of previous studies. Then we considered the interval every 2–3 days or weekly, since its therapeutic effect tends to last for 2–7 days in most patients according to the literature and our initial observations. Maintenance of previous treatments was according to the evaluation of the psychiatrist in charge of the case, but no other medication was introduced simultaneously. Acute effects were assessed 90 min after the first ketamine dose in 11 patients with the question; 'how is your mood right now?' with the possibility of giving a score from 0 to 10. Patients were instructed that 0 corresponds to being very sad/negative/anergic/distressed and 10 corresponds to being cheerful/positive/lively/peaceful.

Results:

Out of 26 patients, 20 achieved remission or clear response for depression, mood instability, cognitive impairment and poor sleep. Three patients had moderate or partial response and three failed to respond. Some patients or their relatives spontaneously used adjectives such as 'sensational', 'amazing', 'incredible' and phrases such as 'I am back to life again' and 'the best night of sleep in years' to describe the observed effects. Many reported to feel potent and confident again, but without the feeling of being under the effects of psychostimulants. No manic, psychotic or dissociative symptoms were observed, but two bipolar patients reported agitation for a few hours. Mild light-headedness was a common but transient side effect, subsiding typically in less than 30 min and more pronounced or present only after the first dose. Eight of the patients reported a clear response after their first dose.

Discussion:

Our clinical observations were that VLDS ketamine produced rapid and robust effects on mood, sleep and cognition in around 75% of patients, with very good tolerability in most cases. The effect on sleep was often reported as remarkable for inducing a deep and repairing sleep, in line with previous findings of increased slow wave sleep by ketamine injection. Also, some patients retained their therapeutic response even after stopping ketamine treatment, which may be associated with the strong neuroplastic changes produced by ketamine, as shown in animal studies, but longer and more systematic observations are necessary.

These therapeutic benefits of VLDS ketamine in most patients with refractory depressive episodes resemble the descriptions of i.v. ketamine, but with better tolerance, ease of use and safety regarding psychiatric adverse events, allowing prolonged and even continuous treatment at home. Regarding clinical safety, no major complications have been reported with ketamine infusion. It is considered safe clinically as an anaesthetic and the effect of repeated treatment in patients with pain have not reported major clinical complications at higher doses than used here.

This is a preliminary exploratory study in a clinical setting with clear limitations. These include the lack of a standardised diagnostic instrument and scales to evaluate psychiatric symptoms and adverse events, the use of unsystematic dose intervals and the inclusion of both unipolar and bipolar patients, many of them with co-morbidities. Thus, the therapeutic effects were evaluated solely on the reports of patients and relatives.

These clinical observations suggest new approaches to design randomised clinical trials, preferably with an active placebo (e.g. benzodiazepine) and evaluating aspects other than depressive symptoms (e.g. mood stability, cognition). If the therapeutic effects are confirmed, VLDS ketamine may become a much more convenient strategy than moderate dose i.v. treatment, allowing its use in a wider range of patients and settings. More studies will also be needed to establish the length of treatment (short term, long term), optimal interval between doses and to better characterise its safety and tolerability.

Examining the details of their patients' illnesses and their previously failed treatments, it is clear that this group were indeed experiencing severe chronic disorders. The self-reported benefits are remarkable given the very low doses used, and it is vital that this study be repeated using a placebo comparison and independent raters. Diogo is in the process of organising an open-label inpatient trial.

When I asked Diogo to tell me about a particularly memorable patient, he replied, 'I cannot recall one special patient. I recall many. What captures my attention is how ketamine restores well-being in general, instead of treating depression only. And with SSRIs, [serotonin reuptake inhibitors, the main group of antidepressants currently being prescribed] for example, we often see personality changes, not always for good, or sometimes family members like that the patient is more passive, but the patient does not feel as her/himself. I love to see patients restoring their cognitive ability to read and how their minds shift from the past to the present and near future. I have seen that in many patients and it's not something that you can capture in the classical scales.'

Diogo continues to use ketamine in clinical practice.

Varun Jaitly

Varun Jaitly is a consultant anaesthetist with an interest in chronic pain. He works at Wrightington, Wigan and Leigh NHS Foundation Trust, which is in the north-west of England.

Of Indian origin, Varun was born in the UK, grew up in the Netherlands, and read medicine at the University of Dundee, Scotland, which awarded him his medical degree (MBChB) in 1989. After working in Scotland for 18 months, he commenced anaesthetic training at Hull. He was subsequently appointed as a registrar on the South Midlands Anaesthetic Rotation Training Scheme (Birmingham) in 1994, where he moved on to do his higher anaesthetic training and which was where he developed an interest in chronic pain. He was appointed as a consultant in 1998.

Varun has lectured and published papers on continuous spinal anaesthesia and the use of ketamine in chronic pain. He also has a professional interest in information technology, having been appointed as the first clinical director in health informatics for the trust in 2005 for a three-year period. As part of his chronic pain commitments, he runs a weekly pain clinic and a weekly injection session. His regular anaesthetic commitments are for trauma/orthopaedics and ENT. Out of hours, he has typical consultant anaesthetist responsibilities for the average English district general hospital.

Varun's importance in the ketamine story became clear in 2013 when he published his account of treating patients suffering from chronic pain with sublingual ketamine over the preceding 13 years.[5] In his paper, he described the treatment results from 32 patients who, in 2012, had been taking ketamine daily for at least the previous 2 years. Apart from the pain relief obtained, he also reviewed the side effects experienced by these patients who (apart from one exception) were taking sublingual ketamine up to three times a day in doses often ranging from 45 mg to 120 mg a day, a typical dose being 90 mg daily.

He explains in his article:

> I came across the 1999 publication by Batchelor[6] where he recounted his experience of using the drug in patients over a period of five years. Shortly after publication of this article, in 2000, I tried ketamine in a patient who had tried all other treatment modalities available to me. The patient reported good pain relief, so I have continued to try other patients with this drug over the years. As I routinely collect outcome data for all my patients using the Pain Audit Collection System database, I decided after several years to evaluate outcomes of patients who have been through my service and tried ketamine. After this initial evaluation and following the reports of ketamine-induced ulcerative

cystitis, I then created a bespoke simple database to allow me to systematically track who had received ketamine and how they had fared as part of a continuous audit process. As there is a dearth of information regarding long-term outcome data in patients who use ketamine as an adjunct in their management of chronic pain, I hope this paper will shed some light on this neglected area of study.

In his paper, Varun details his treatment process:

Ketamine administration:

After appropriate counselling in the outpatients (where patients are given a patient information leaflet and are informed that ketamine is also known as a drug of misuse, a date-rape drug, a dance floor drug, a horse anaesthetic and a human anaesthetic which might make them hallucinate and has a poor success rate in the management of chronic pain), patients are listed for a trial of oral ketamine (technically it is sublingual administration, but it is easier for everyone to say the word 'oral' rather than 'sublingual'). As patients have access to the Internet these days, I feel they are better off hearing this information from me rather than reading about it online and then possibly feeling that I was hiding this information from them. Most patients are considered to be eligible for consideration for ketamine treatment. Patients with a history of substance misuse and female patients of childbearing age who are yet to complete their family are not usually offered this treatment modality.

Patients who wish to try ketamine are asked to attend the Day Surgical Unit (DSU) on the day that I carry out my injection list. The ketamine is administered prior to starting the injection list. If possible, patients are admitted to a quiet side room on our DSU. I ask patients to take all their regular painkillers as normal (so I can judge better the interaction between these drugs and the ketamine). Prior to asking a patient to sign their 'NHS Informed Consent Form' I ask the patient to numerically rate their pain score (0–10) and I make a note of this. I then administer the sublingual ketamine (Pfizer Limited, Sandwich, Kent CT13 9NJ, UK). It is the intravenous preparation that I use. For many years it has been the 100 mg/ml preparation that has been used but, more recently, manufacturing has been relocated and stocks are running low (personal communication from pharmacy) so currently we have been using the 50 mg/ml preparation. The usual dose is 20 mg and I ask the patient to hold it sublingually as long as they can, and inform them that they can swallow if they feel they are going to drown in their own saliva. After completing my injection list I return to review the patient. I ask the patient if they have had any benefit and ask them to numerically rate their pain score again on the same 0–10 scale. It is clearly easier to judge the utility of the ketamine if the pain is constant rather than episodic.

Patients are asked to complete a ketamine treatment agreement if they appear to have found the ketamine helpful. One copy of the agreement is given to the patient and the other is filed in the medical records. I ask patients to demonstrate using tap water that they can successfully draw up and self-administer the correct amount of drug before discharge. Patients are given a 30 day supply of ketamine in a standard NHS drug-dispensing bottle (the shelf life of ketamine in this bottle is only 30 days—personal communication from Trust pharmacist). The usual dose suggested to the patient is 20 mg to be taken three times per day via the sublingual route. Patients are advised that they can experiment a little with the dose but to not exceed the total daily dose of 60 mg per day. Suitable dose options could be 30 mg twice a day or a single maximum dose of 40 mg, with the remaining 20 mg either split into two doses of 10 mg, or one dose of 20 mg. Patients are requested to self-assess which dose regime appears to suit them and they are reviewed in the clinic four weeks later. If the ketamine is still helping at this stage, patients are initially reviewed again at three months, and if all is well at that point, patients are then reviewed on a six-monthly basis and repeated prescriptions issued at each outpatient visit. The medication is dispensed by the hospital pharmacy on a monthly basis.

Varun's analysis of his results showed that 20% of those patients who tried the initial dose of ketamine experienced sufficient benefit to warrant continuation therapy.

As quoted from his paper below, he raises a number of important issues in his discussion section:

Discussion:

Although the randomised controlled trial is the gold standard experimental design for testing a novel intervention, many areas of clinically important knowledge are best, or most efficiently, informed by high-quality observational data. I make no claim to have provided randomised controlled information or evidence in this paper—I have merely written about what I have observed when my patients have tried sublingual ketamine in an attempt to help them manage their pain. This data therefore comes with all the warnings and caveats that apply to this type of information.

Anyone thinking about prescribing ketamine in the way that I have needs to answer for themselves the following questions:

Does ketamine work?
Is it safe?
How do I use it?

This data suggests that about 1 in 5 patients seem to get some sort of benefit from ketamine in the long term. There is clearly a huge placebo effect and this is manifest by the number of patients who abandon treatment within the first few years of trying the drug. It is argued that the 1 in 5 patients who appear to have a long-lasting response to ketamine are also demonstrating a placebo response (Wells, C., communication on pain consultants Google group). While this may be the case, I would point out that the same patients did not elicit the same remarkably persisting 'placebo' response when they tried other evidence-based drugs like amitriptyline, duloxetine, gabapentin or pregabalin beforehand.

When patients did report benefit, the average pain relief that patients reported was calculated to be 50–60%. However, the benefit reported does not appear to translate itself in the form of better BPI [Brief Pain Inventory] scores. Eyeballing the data does not show any clear pattern or trend with respect to pain scores or interference with various elements of the BPI. The question therefore that has to be asked is that if ketamine is not improving BPI, what is it really doing?

It is possible that ketamine may be improving the low mood, which often accompanies patients who have chronic pain. There is randomised controlled evidence that intravenous ketamine can act as an acute antidepressant with effects that appear to persist long after the drug is considered to have cleared from the body.

I have considered the possibility that the effect seen is due to this small group of patients having become physically dependent on ketamine. On the other hand, patients who abandoned ketamine therapy within the first two years did not report an abstinence syndrome. Anecdotally, over the years, patients who have been on treatment longer than two years occasionally run out of ketamine and sometimes have to wait a few days before having the medication dispensed. To the best of my knowledge, these patients have also not reported an abstinence syndrome, although they do report their pain gets worse. In conclusion, it is unlikely that physical dependence has occurred.

The lack of long-term safety data for a drug such as ketamine has been of concern to some authors. The limited data I present appears to show that at low doses there does not appear to be any easily observable harm stemming from the use of ketamine. Currently, the total daily dose for most of my patients does not tend to exceed 120 mg per day, with the odd exception. There is evidence to suggest that liver and urinary tract side effects are dose-dependent phenomena. This is reassuring—after all, we still use paracetamol for pain relief, even though we know that in overdose, the side effects can be serious. There is also data to suggest that high doses of ketamine may actually cause hyperalgesia, so there are several reasons to not escalate the dose of ketamine.

My data suggests that hallucinations are not that common at the dose used. If they do occur, they are not usually too intrusive, although one patient had to decrease her dose to 1 mg three times per day. Higher doses made her very sleepy and even on this lower dose she would experience some visual disturbances (e.g. the ceiling looked like syrup, which would drip to the floor). This patient discontinued her treatment after almost two years after not attending for follow-up. Another elderly patient saw an apparition of her deceased mother standing at the bottom of her hospital bed when she tried ketamine for the first time. This was clearly unsettling for her because her mother had passed away many years ago. Needless to say, this patient did not progress to taking ketamine on a regular basis. Another regular user of ketamine reported that once, after having taken ketamine on an empty stomach, and subsequently having breakfast, that his breakfast cereal looked like rocks.

It is argued that if the beneficial effect of ketamine is a placebo effect, then there is clearly an opportunity cost associated with my activity. On the other hand, if this is a placebo effect, this 'placebo' effect has satisfied my patients for a considerable period of time and I have helped my patients to avoid some of the riskier interventions that we pain physicians have at our disposal and that they may not necessarily have wanted to pursue.

Unfortunately, there does not appear to be a consistent pattern as to what types of pain ketamine is most helpful for. Some would argue that snake oil appears to have similar breadth of beneficial effect.

Some proponents of ketamine prefer the use of an intravenous infusion approach, rather than the sublingual approach. In 2012, Patil and colleagues published a five year retrospective analysis of 49 patients with chronic pain who had undergone a total of 369 outpatient ketamine infusions between them. They concluded that 'in patients with severe refractory pain of multiple aetiologies, subanaesthetic ketamine infusions may improve Visual Analogue Scale scores'. In half of their patients, relief lasted for up to three weeks with minimal side effects. Some advocates of ketamine have gone even further and used substantial doses of ketamine to induce a coma in an attempt to 'reboot' the central nervous system, but death is a rare complication of this procedure—hence my preference for using the sublingual route at a fraction of these doses.

He concludes, 'The long-term use of low-dose sublingual ketamine in chronic pain appears to be safe. Some patients find it very helpful for their pain when other drugs have not worked. To date, using it long term has not appeared to cause too many problems.'

Those who have concerns about the hazards of using ketamine over extended periods should read this paper in its entirety. Varun has shown that many of our fears about causing unacceptable side effects or contributing to abuse or addiction through medical treatment are unwarranted.

Varun continues to prescribe ketamine, and one of his patients has now been taking it daily for 18 years. He is currently working to develop a system for evaluating ketamine responses and side effects that can be used to gather information internationally.

Other Ketamine Doctors

The following details were obtained from the Ketamine Advocacy Network:

Dr Nancy Sajben
Doctor: Dr Nancy Sajben, MD
Address: 9834 Genesee Avenue, La Jolla, CA 92037
Specialty: neurology
Treatment type: intranasal
Adjuncts: oxytocin, low-dose naltrexone
Phone: 858-622-0500
http://painsandiego.com/tag/ketamine

Interventional Psychiatry Associates
Doctor: Dr Terrence Early, MD
Address: 1913 State Street, Santa Barbara, CA 93110
Specialty: psychiatry
Treatment type: IV infusion
Phone: 805-845-8770
www.ipasb.com

Portland Ketamine Clinic
Doctor: Dr Enrique Abreu, MD
Address: Portland, OR
Specialty: anaesthesiology
Treatment type: IV infusion
www.portlandketamineclinic.com

Ketamine Treatment Centers of Princeton
Doctor: Dr. Steven P. Levine, MD / Martin Bier, MD
Address: 800 Bunn Drive, Suite 304, Princeton, NJ 08540
Specialty: Psychiatry
Treatment type: IV infusion
Phone: 888-566-8774
Note: Click the link above, then select the Princeton, NJ location

New York Ketamine Infusions
Doctor: Dr Glen Brooks, MD
Address: 80 Maiden Lane, New York, NY 10038
Specialty: anaesthesiology
Treatment type: IV infusion
Adjuncts: Nuedexta
Notes: For some patients, oral ketamine may be prescribed after
    initial infusions
Phone: 917-261-7370
nyketamine.com

References

1. Angelo De Gioannis, Diego De Leo, 'Managing Suicidal Patients in Clinical Practice', *Open Journal of Psychiatry*, 2 (January 2012), 49–60. <http://dx.doi.org/10.4236/ojpsych.2012.21008>

2. A. De Gioannis, D. De Leo, 'Oral Ketamine Augmentation for Chronic Suicidality in Treatment-Resistant Depression', Australian and New Zealand Journal of Psychiatry. 48/7 (22 January 2014), 686.

3. ABC 7:30 report Tracy Bowden 21/01/15.

4. Diogo R. Lara, Luisa W. Bisol, and Luciano R. Munari, 'Antidepressant, Mood Stabilizing and Procognitive Effects of Very Low Dose Sublingual Ketamine in Refractory Unipolar and Bipolar Depression', *International Journal of Neuropsychopharmacology*, 16 (2013), 2111–2117. DOI:10.1017/S1461145713000485.

5. V. K. Jaitly, 'Sublingual Ketamine in Chronic Pain: Service Evaluation by Examining More Than 200 Patient Years of Data', *Journal of Observational Pain Medicine*, 1/2 (2013). The content of this chapter which relates to Dr Jaitly's contribution to our knowledge of ketamine has largely been transcribed from his original open-access article, which was distributed under the terms of the Creative Commons Attribution License, which permits unrestricted use, distribution, and reproduction in any medium, provided the original work is properly cited.

6. 'Chronic Pain Control', *Health Technology Assessment*, 1/6 (1997), i–iv; 1–135. 11. Batchelor, G. 'Ketamine in Neuropathic Pain', *Pain Society Newsletter*, 1/7 (1999), 19.

Chapter 8

Who Should Try It?
Who Should Not?

To decide who should try ketamine treatment for depression, we need to draw up a risk–benefit equation for each patient. The patients for whom, in my view, the balance tilts clearly to the 'try' side are those patients in palliative care suffering from pain, anxiety, and depression. In this situation, the priority is to use fast-acting, effective treatments with as few side effects as possible and any concerns about potential long-term side effects are irrelevant. Ketamine can be given by simple non-invasive routes (e.g. oral, sublingual, and intranasal), and it combines well with other agents—e.g. opiates, which are commonly used for symptom relief in this setting.

Secondly, there are those patients who are acutely suicidal. There have now been a number of studies pointing to a rapid reduction in suicidal thinking—in some, even when there has been no clear lift in mood. This is a very important issue as an effective treatment in this situation can enable a broader range of choices in a very stressful situation. For example, instead of needing to be hospitalised, patients can be cared for in less-restrictive settings and not be taken away from their usual supports. Given that being in a hospital is not in itself a barrier to suicide, ketamine can also be used in inpatient wards. By prescribing ketamine, doctors can gain breathing space during which more extensive help can be mobilised. Most importantly, the use of ketamine needs to be seen as a starting point for intensive treatment, not as an answer in itself.

Global suicide rates in the last 12 months have been estimated at one million[1]

In the USA, suicide rates have remained stable but have been persistently high for the past 20 years at 41,000 per year. Each year, more than 1 million adults attempt suicide, and 17% of teens seriously consider suicide; 70% of suicide deaths are among white males. Here in Australia, an estimated 2,500 people suicide each year.

Reistaler et al. in 2015 summarised the studies on ketamine and suicidality:[2]

ABSTRACT:

To review the published literature on the efficacy of ketamine for the treatment of suicidal ideation (SI). The PubMed and Cochrane databases were searched up to January 2015 for clinical trials and case reports describing therapeutic ketamine administration to patients presenting with SI/suicidality. Searches were also conducted for relevant background material regarding the pharmacological function of ketamine. Nine publications (six studies and three case reports) met the search criteria for assessing SI after administration of sub anaesthetic ketamine. There were no studies examining the effect on suicide attempts or death by suicide. Each study demonstrated a rapid and clinically significant reduction in SI, with results similar to previously described data on ketamine and treatment-resistant depression. A total of 137 patients with SI have been reported in the literature as receiving therapeutic ketamine. Seven studies delivered a dose of 0.5 mg/kg intravenously over 40 min, while one study administered a 0.2 mg/kg intravenous bolus and another study administered a liquid suspension. The earliest significant results were seen after 40 min, and the longest results were observed up to 10 days post infusion. Consistent with clinical research on ketamine as a rapid and effective treatment for depression, ketamine has shown early preliminary evidence of a reduction in depressive symptoms, as well as reducing SI, with minimal short-term side effects.

Additional studies are needed to further investigate its mechanism of action, long-term outcomes, and long-term adverse effects (including abuse) and benefits.

More recent work on ketamine and suicide can be found in Chapter 9.

Ketamine Reduces Suicidal Thoughts

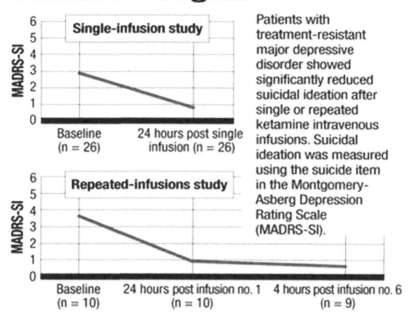

Patients with treatment-resistant major depressive disorder showed significantly reduced suicidal ideation after single or repeated ketamine intravenous infusions. Suicidal ideation was measured using the suicide item in the Montgomery-Asberg Depression Rating Scale (MADRS-SI).

Source: Rebecca Price, M.D., et al., *Biological Psychiatry*, September 1, 2009

Other patients for whom a trial of ketamine is warranted are those suffering from treatment-resistant depression. This is the group which has been most widely studied over the past 18 years, and given the high mortality rate of these patients [in the USA, on average they will die 20 years earlier than their peers], it is my view that the potential benefits of ketamine therapy greatly outweigh the risks. We know that a third of depressed patients do not respond at all to our current medications and psychotherapies and that a third respond only in part. This leaves a large number of people who could benefit from a trial of ketamine. In addition, it would be far better to use ketamine as part of professional clinical care than to leave people to vote with their feet and seek to obtain the drug illegally. The example of the widespread and growing use of self-prescribed 'medical' marijuana shows us clearly that people in pain, both physical and mental, will go to great lengths seek relief.

In an article in the *Psychiatric Times* in 2014, Allen Francis talked to Dr Weiden, who is a professor of psychiatry at the University of Illinois Medical Centre and has spent his professional career working on improving outcomes and reducing side effects and complications for people with serious mental illnesses.[3]

Dr Weiden explained that in the USA, life expectancy had increased from 70 years in the 1970s to 80 years at present, most probably related to the decline in smoking.

Certain groups (e.g. black Americans) live for 5 years less, but one group suffers by far the most with an average of 20 years of reduced life, this being similar to the life expectancy in Third World countries. This is the group diagnosed with serious mental illnesses—schizophrenia, bipolar disorder, and treatment-resistant depression.

We have known for many years that individuals with serious mental illnesses are more likely to have medical problems (such as diabetes, hypertension, or heart disease), but most of the mortality concern was focussed on the risk of suicide and other kinds of injuries that come from poorly controlled psychiatric symptoms.

However, it became clear in 2006 when a new study of mortality statistics showed that individuals with chronic mental illnesses were dying between 13 and 31 years early, averaging to over 20 years of life lost relative to age-matched general populations. Their causes of death were the same causes of death as in the general population, only happening on average about 20 years earlier. Thus patients were dying in their fifties from conditions such as diabetes, heart disease, respiratory illness, and cancer, which would not kill their peers till 20 years later.

The causes as always are complex, with patients experiencing chronic mental illness less likely to eat well, to exercise, to seek timely care for common ailments and more likely to smoke and be more non-compliant with treatment. In addition, they have higher rates of death from injury, accidents, homicide, and suicide. Those taking either no medication or very high doses are the most vulnerable.

What other group in society would tolerate such inequality?

When we examine more closely the numbers of people who are affected worldwide by depressive disorders, the challenge of delivering effective treatment is massive.

> Depression is an increasingly common debilitating illness, currently projected to affect 121 million people worldwide by 2020 (World Health Organisation, 2012).
>
> Serious depressive states, whether unipolar or bipolar, have a lifetime prevalence of 15–20%, and are projected to become the second leading cause of disability worldwide by 2020.[4]
>
> The global economic loss due to depression, anxiety, bipolar disorder and PTSD is estimated at $1300 billion annually and the global sales of medications to treat these disorders each year is $50 billion.[5]
>
> Australia, with a population of 23 million currently has 3 million people suffering from depression and/or anxiety disorders. The estimated cost to the economy is $20 billion each year.[6]
>
> Every year, 14.8 million Americans suffer from major depression. Of those who seek treatment, 30% to 40% will not get better or fully recover with standard medication and counselling approaches. That puts them at greater risk of alcohol and drug abuse, suicide attempts and significantly shortens life expectancy.[7]

Next, there are those who have been helped by our standard treatments but who experience high levels of unwanted side effects (e.g. sexual dysfunction, weight gain, sleep difficulties, and problems with thinking and memory). Many so afflicted either stop their medication or reduce it to less-effective levels. In addition, for some patients, our psychotherapies are too expensive and time consuming. It is possible that adding low-dose ketamine in the short term could assist in both these situations as it does not induce the same side effects and there is evidence that it enhances the benefits of standard medications; those in psychotherapy may respond more quickly when brief augmentation with ketamine enhances the therapy.

More contentious would be using ketamine for patients needing a more rapid resolution of depressive symptoms for personal or financial reasons, e.g. someone whose relationship is failing as a consequence of their mood state or someone who cannot afford to take time off work to recover. Ketamine-enhanced standard medication and psychotherapy could be considered in these situations.

Finally, there are those who have benefited from taking ketamine in the past and are desperately seeking relief.

> This.can.help 2014:
>
> I have bipolar 2 (and all the associated neurological aches and ailments that accompany it), social anxiety disorder, ADD, depression, generalised anxiety, PMDD, and all-around awfulness.
>
> Zoloft was my first script, and, after 3 days passed out exhausted, and 2 more weeks of blah, I actually felt really good! It didn't last, though, and higher doses caused mania. I stopped taking it, and was prescribed Depakote—worst thing I had ever experienced. I felt like I was being smashed into the earth by unseen forces. I stopped taking that, of course.
>
> Around the same time, I discovered low-dose intranasal ketamine therapy on my own (before the disastrous re-classification of the drug in 1999). Suddenly, no other medications were needed! It was A MIRACLE. Except it was one I couldn't discuss with anyone and be taken seriously.
>
> I had 3.5 brilliant, successful, happy, healthy years without any negative side-effects, increase in use, or physiological dependency or withdrawal, or any other complications; the drug became unavailable (and unjustly vilified); and I have spent the last 15 years with many doctors and dozens of FDA approved meds—some helped briefly, others caused HORRIFYING side-effects.
>
> I know there are doctors in NYC who are prescribing low-dose nasal spray infusions. I am desperate to find them. I have a great deal of knowledge and experience that should be very enlightening for ANYONE genuinely interested in HELPING us. If anyone knows ethical doctors out there who are willing to listen and learn and help save lives, PLEASE, PLEASE respond here. I am dreadfully afraid that my life will fall apart. I do not have the money for IV infusions NOR

do I think they are necessary or the best way to do this (at least for me). Health insurance doesn't pay for any of this, but an inhaler, or two, a month would be doable, and life saving.[8]

I will explore other ketamine-responsive conditions apart from depression more fully in the next chapter.

Other patients who have not benefitted from standard care (i.e. proper trials of psychotherapy and medications and where there is some evidence of efficacy) include those with OCD, PTSD, anxiety disorders, and eating disorders. Given that many patients with depression suffer also from these conditions (co-morbidity), ketamine therapy becomes an attractive option.

There are some conditions where there have been a few positive case reports of ketamine treatment, including autism and intermittent explosive disorder. In the physical realm, apart from ketamine's use in anaesthesia and pain medicine, there are also a number of conditions for which ketamine has shown to be beneficial. These include asthma, epilepsy, and traumatic brain injury, priapism and L-dopa induced dyskinesia.

Although none of the following findings would in itself be a reason to try or not to try ketamine, there is some evidence emerging from trials suggesting that certain patients are more likely to respond. These include women, those with a personal or family history of alcohol abuse, the overweight, those with a particular genetic enzyme variant (val-val), those with small hippocampi (a brain area serving memory and orientation), those with a specific blood fatty acid profile, and patients showing slower pretreatment processing speed.

Who should not?

There are very few absolute contraindications to trying ketamine, but there are certain groups who will require more intensive monitoring.

- Those allergic to ketamine: This is very rare. A recent literature survey showed that 4 probable allergic reactions have been reported over the past 50 years.
- Cardiovascular instability, particularly uncontrolled high blood pressure: Ketamine may be safer than alternatives but would require cautious dosing and a high level of supervision.
- Liver and kidney failure: In the context of palliative care, ketamine may still be helpful.

- Current psychosis: Patients with melancholia (a severe depressive illness with excessive guilt being prominent) and psychotic depression have been successfully treated with ketamine. Also, patients with the diagnosis of schizophrenia who took part in ketamine trials in the 1990s did not experience lasting harm. Bipolar youths with a history of psychotic symptoms responded well to ketamine.[9] Ketamine is increasingly being used to treat excited delirium, usually a drug-induced psychotic state. Given that an estimated 50% of patients with the diagnosis of schizophrenia also experience depressive symptoms and that our standard antidepressants are not proven to be helpful in this group and that the suicide rate is 5%, both ECT and ketamine treatment are possible options.
- Current addiction: Ketamine has been successfully used as part of treatment programs for heroin, cocaine and alcohol dependence. There is one positive study of ketamine use for a current benzodiazepine addict taking 15 mg of lorazepam daily.[10] Anecdotally, however, doctors wonder whether taking benzodiazepines during ketamine treatment can blunt the response to ketamine.
- In pregnancy, safety is not established: As of 2014, the FDA has not formally assigned ketamine to a pregnancy category. Animal studies at higher-than-human doses failed to reveal evidence of teratogenicity or impairment of fertility. There is no controlled data in human pregnancy. Since the safe use in pregnancy and delivery has not been established, the manufacturer recommends that ketamine be considered contraindicated in pregnant women.[11] Briggs et al. have assigned Ketamine to pregnancy Risk Factor B as probably compatible.[12]
- Australia's category B3: 'Drugs which have been taken by only a limited number of pregnant women and women of childbearing age, without an increase in the frequency of malformation or other direct or indirect harmful effects on the human foetus having been observed. Studies in animals have shown evidence of an increased occurrence of foetal damage, the significance of which is considered uncertain in humans.'[13]
- Ketamine breastfeeding warnings: There are no data on the excretion of ketamine into human milk. However, because

ketamine is a general anaesthetic agent, breastfeeding would not be possible while using the drug. According to Briggs et al., ketamine should be undetectable in maternal plasma approximately 11 hours after a dose. Nursing after this time should not expose the infant to significant amounts of the drug. (This does not examine ketamine metabolites.)

- Closed-angle glaucoma: There is a small risk of increased intraocular pressure.

References

1. Ketamine Advocacy Network. <www.ketamineadvocacynetwork. org/>.
2. Lael Reinstatler, Nagy A. Youssef, 'Ketamine as a Potential Treatment for Suicidal Ideation: A Systematic Review of the Literature', *Drugs in R&D*, 15 (10 February 2015), 37–43. DOI 10.1007/s40268-015-0081-0.
3. Allen Francis, *Psychiatric Times*. <http://www.psychiatric times.com/severe-mental-illness-means-dying-young#sthash. Z532fydf.dpuf>.
4. Global Health Statistics (Murray and Lopez 1996).
5. Ketamine Advocacy Network. www.ketamineadvocacynetwork.org/
6. From the feed 6/4/15 SBS-2.
7. *Archives of General Psychiatry*, 62/6 (June 2015): 617–27.
8. Ketamine Advocacy Network. www.ketamineadvocacynetwork.org/
9. Demitri F. Papolos, Martin H. Teicher, Gianni L. Faedda, Patricia Murphy, Steven Mattis, 'Clinical Experience Using Intranasal Ketamine in the Treatment of Pediatric Bipolar Disorder/Fear of Harm Phenotype', 2012 Elsevier B. V.
10. M. Liebrenz, R. Stohler, A. Borgeat, 'Repeated Intravenous Ketamine Therapy in a Patient with Treatment-Resistant Major Depression', *World Journal of Biological Psychiatry*; 10/4 Pt 2 (2009), 640–3.
11. 'Ketamine Pregnancy and Breastfeeding Warnings'. <drugs.com>.
12. Briggs et al., *Drugs in Pregnancy and Lactation* (4th edn).
13. Ketamine Datasheet Sep 10, Medsafe. <www.medsafe.govt.nz/ profs/datasheet/k/ketamineinf.pdf>.

Chapter 9

Other Conditions Treated
with Ketamine

In this chapter, we will examine the use of ketamine in a range of other psychiatric and physical disorders. Given that few patients suffer from a single illness, it is encouraging to see that the use of ketamine is being explored so widely. For some of these conditions, the use of ketamine has been described in just one case report, but others have been more widely investigated.

Most randomised trials exclude patients who have co-morbid conditions, are suicidal, or do not choose to volunteer, so they are not the patients we usually see in our daily work. In the more comprehensive STAR*D trial, around 80% of their patients had co-morbid conditions and were suicidal, which would have excluded them from the standard randomised trials, and these patients had significantly lower responses and remission rates. So real-life patients are sicker and harder to help.[1]

In terms of ongoing research into ketamine, there are 671 clinical trials currently recorded on the clinical trials.gov website.

Of the 222 active studies being conducted in the domain of psychiatry, 117 are investigating the use of ketamine for the treatment of major depressive disorder, 22 for suicidality and 83 for various anxiety disorders.

In psychiatry, other conditions in which ketamine has been used include:

- autism
- rett syndrome
- intermittent explosive disorder
- generalised anxiety disorder
- obsessive-compulsive disorder
- social anxiety disorder
- post-traumatic stress disorder
- suicidal thinking
- alcoholism and heroin addiction
- cocaine dependence
- eating disorders
- borderline disorder
- depression with psychosis

Autism

Drugs such as memantine and D-cycloserine that also work on the glutamate system have been trialled in autism.

Logan K. Wink, MD, reported on a case study of a 29-year-old patient with autism spectrum disorder, major depressive disorder, anorexia nervosa, and obsessive-compulsive disorder.[2]

Over the previous 15 years, she had been extensively treated with medications, hospitalisation, and ECT. She was chronically suicidal.

She was given intranasal ketamine in addition to her current medications, selegiline, lamotrigine, naltrexone, and clonazepam. She showed improvement within 24 hours of her first and succeeding doses of ketamine, with a lift in mood, improved interaction with others, a decrease in her urge to purge, a higher tolerance to changes in routine, and increased energy and concentration. Notably, the length of time spent looking at facial expressions on a visual tracking test, one measure of autistic behaviour, also improved through the study. She experienced short-term dizziness and headaches after the treatments, and there were no changes in her vital signs. The broad clinical improvement reported is interesting, and a progress report from Dr Wink would be very helpful.

Rett Syndrome

Rett syndrome is a rare genetic neurological disorder of the grey matter of the brain caused by mutations in the gene MECP2. There is no known treatment, but funding has now been received for a full-scale study using ketamine.

In an interview in the *Rare Disease Report*, Monica Coenraads, the executive director of the Rett Syndrome Research Trust, explained that the trust had provided the funds as there had been numerous anecdotal reports of children improving after receiving ketamine for medical and dental procedures.

In addition, studies in mice models of Rett syndrome by Dr Katz and colleagues had shown improvements in brain function and breathing following the administration of ketamine.[3]

Intermittent Explosive Disorder

Ketamine is used to sedate violent and agitated patients in emergency departments. J. E. Berner gave an account of its use in a patient experiencing long-term difficulty with anger control.[4]

His patient was 20 years old and had a lifelong history of rage attack episodes two to three times a day, which was becoming more problematic as he grew older and stronger. The attacks were triggered by denial of repeated inappropriate requests and were often followed by guilt and regret with suicidal gestures. In his late teens, parental injury and police involvement as often as twice a week was common.

He had a history of prenatal stroke with subsequent brain damage and epilepsy. Over the years, he had been unsuccessfully trialled on seven anticonvulsants, six antidepressants, four antipsychotics, and many other agents, including lithium.

After an emergency room visit at age 18 years resulted in an involuntary treatment referral, the patient's family provided consent for a trial of ketamine. Over the next 16 months, doses of intranasal ketamine up to 60 mg over four hours, taken when required, generally kept the rages under control. Tolerability was excellent, and the initial prompting by the patient's parents for him to take ketamine was later followed by him spontaneously requesting a dose. Cumulative doses greater than 200 mg/day, however, produced hallucinosis.

Generalised Anxiety disorder

A study by Paul Glue et al using ketamine given subcutaneously appeared in the April 2017 edition of the Journal of Psychopharmacology entitled
"Ketamine's dose related effects on anxiety symptoms in patients with treatment-refractory anxiety disorders." [15]

12 patients with generalised anxiety disorder and/or social anxiety disorder, who were not currently depressed, were given ketamine subcutaneously at ascending levels of 0.25, 0.5, and 1.0mg/kg bodyweight weekly for 3 weeks.
10 of the 12 showed rapid improvement that persisted for 3-7 days at the higher doses.
Two patients experienced nausea and two had dissociative symptoms at the higher doses.
These patients had been ill for an average of 6 years, had not responded well to standard therapy and were highly comorbid - 10 had been diagnosed with generalised anxiety disorder [GAD], 9 had social anxiety disorder [SAD], 5 had panic disorder [PD], 2 post-traumatic stress disorder [PTSD] and 11 had a past history of major depression.

As Glue commented, these results suggest that ketamine can be beneficial for a range of negative emotional states. There have been prior positive results in trials of patients who were given ketamine for obsessive-compulsive disorder [OCD] and PTSD. There are also similarities in the disruptions to brain circuits shown in anxiety and depressive disorders.

Glue et al then went on to explore how those members of the trial group who had experienced a short-term response to ketamine fared with maintenance treatment over a 3 month period.16 This was an open label, uncontrolled trial.
21 of the 25 patients entering the initial trial had been responders and 18 completed the maintenance phase.

20 patients received subcutaneous ketamine 1.0mg/kg bodyweight injected at one or two weekly intervals. Most [16] received treatment weekly.

Diagnostically 15 patients were diagnosed with GAD, 18 SAD and 4 PD with the mean duration of anxiety symptoms being 13.9 years. At one hour post injection an average 50% reduction was noted on anxiety rating scales.

Dissociative symptoms were transient and reduced over the time of the study.

The most significant finding was that all 18 completers reported improved work and social function. Most of the patients who responded to the initial treatment remained in remission throughout the 3 months maintenance phase.

The most common transient side effects were nausea, dizziness, and blurred vision. One patient had temporary blood pressure elevation thought likely to be due to inadvertent intravenous administration of ketamine.

After 3 months when ketamine therapy was ceased 5 patients remained well, 8 experienced a partial relapse and 5 a full relapse within 2 weeks of the last dose.

These studies indicate that ketamine therapy can be helpful for a range of anxiety disorders and that this efficacy can be maintained for months with ongoing treatment with most side effects decreasing over time. These have been uncontrolled trials, but the results of a midazolam-controlled investigation are due shortly. The group is also investigating EEG changes recorded during therapy looking for potential biomarkers predicting response.

Also in regard to generalised anxiety disorder [GAD] J Singh and Daly, in a letter to JAMA in May 2018 confirmed that they had analysed GAD data taken from a phase 2 trial of intranasal esketamine for depression.[19] They reported a significant improvement in symptom scores following administration of 84 mg of intranasal esketamine. This was apparent one week after the initial treatment and was sustained during the 9 weeks of the open label phase of the study during which patients received repeated doses of esketamine.

Obsessive-Compulsive Disorder

After reading the next paper, I decided to start trialling ketamine, first for a patient with OCD, then for other treatment-resistant conditions.

In 2013 lead author Carolyn Rodriguez (MD, PhD, assistant professor at Columbia University in New York) presented the results of a trial using intravenous ketamine at 0.5 mg/kg body weight for a small group of patients who were unmedicated and suffering from OCD without co-morbid depression.[5] The trial, although involving only 15 patients, was randomised, double-blind, and placebo-controlled with a crossover period of at least 1 week between the injections. Saline placebo was used. Patients had not responded to at least one previous trial of therapy and had near-constant obsessive thoughts.

Half the patients responded, showing a minimum 35% reduction of symptoms on the Yale–Brown Obsessive-Compulsive Scale, this change beginning mid infusion and being sustained for at least a week. Two weeks after the ketamine infusion, 40% were still recorded as responders.

Positive patients' comments included the following: 'I feel as if the weight of OCD has been lifted . . . I want to feel this way forever', 'I feel like someone is giving me an explanation [for my OCD]', 'I don't have any intrusive thoughts. I was laughing when you couldn't find the key, which normally is a trigger for me. This is amazing, unbelievable. This is right out of a movie', 'I tried to have OCD thoughts, but I couldn't'.

Given that most patients with OCD respond slowly, if at all, to standard medications, usually taking 6–10 weeks to experience a 50% reduction in symptoms, to achieve such a result for some with a single infusion is very encouraging. There are currently five trials planned or in progress, examining ketamine's role in the treatment of OCD.

Social Anxiety Disorder

In the USA, there is one trial under way for patients suffering from social anxiety disorder. The following account comes from Govinda on a social anxiety forum online on the eleventh of August two thousand and fourteen.

Just Tried Ketamine Infusion:[6]

It was a bit hard to find, but I was eventually pointed in the direction of someone who could give me a ketamine infusion as a possible treatment for anxiety/depression. I corresponded with someone at a University doing a study, but in the end it was just my psychiatrist telling me about a particular anaesthesiologist who was willing to perform it. The psych only gave out this info after a lot of badgering and was very sceptical. But I had done a fair amount of research and had to know.

Basically, I found that it helped depression greatly and anxiety in more of a roundabout way. The first few days afterwards I felt calm, clear, and like everything was less heavy and awful. Problems were still problems, but they seemed workable. And it helped in terms of social anxiety because, since I was more enthusiastic about life in general, I was more talkative, probably noticed less judgement in the faces of others, and felt just generally more confident. Also, I felt mentally sharper and articulated things more clearly. That feeling began to fade, as I assumed from reading it would, after a few days—a great few days.

But . . . I can't afford it. It was $ 450 for a 40 minute infusion of 0.5 mg/kg body weight. From what I've seen, some of the most successful protocols call for this being done 3x in the 1st week, then at least a couple times a month after that. Relapse times varied a lot in what I saw. My insurance company not surprisingly won't touch it—though I've heard of people winning over certain carriers for ketamine for other off-label uses.

There are companies that are trying to get analogues approved, for example glyx-13 is in stage 2 or 3 clinical trials, but, as most of you know, that may take forever, may not have the same effects, or may never see the light of day at all.

I had to know though. And I'm glad I tried; maybe if I'm better off financially and still suffering in the future I'll give it a true, long-term shot. Just for a fuller picture, I should say that, in the days leading up to the infusion I had been feeling suicidally bad, and was using pregabalin, klonopin, and a very low dose of an maoi—one of many, many cocktails I've tried over the last 12 years.

This is a follow-up post on 14/11/2014:

Actually, scratch that bit about needing to be ultra-rich in order to take ketamine for anxiety + depression. If you go the infusion route, then yes, it is expensive. But I'm finding more and more that individuals are getting sublingual and intranasal formulations for chronic pain syndrome—that still wouldn't be covered by insurance, but it would leave out the equipment, anaesthesiologist, nurse and other fees that really jack up the price.

Now the new challenge: finding someone to prescribe. Well, I overcame it last time, so I have some confidence.

Taylor et al in 2017 examined the effect of ketamine on symptoms in patients diagnosed with social anxiety disorder. [17]This was a small crossover study enrolling 18 patients who were given a single dose of intravenous ketamine 0.5mg/kg bodyweight versus a saline placebo with doses given 28 days apart to avoid carryover effects. 6 of the 18 completers responded.

There was no observed effect on concurrent mild to moderate depressive symptoms and the treatment was well tolerated.

Compared to the Glue study there was a lesser, though more durable, effect obtained with increased social engagement being reported.

Post-Traumatic Stress Disorder

With ketamine's tradition of use for anaesthesia and pain relief in war zones, it is no surprise to see interest in its efficacy for the treatment of post-traumatic stress disorder (PTSD).

There had been reports that ketamine given during surgery for burns soldiers sustained in Afghanistan and Iraq had the unexpected benefit of reducing the incidence of PTSD by 50% compared to those who were treated with other anaesthetics.

The army has supported further research into treatment of PTSD, this time using intranasal ketamine and comparing it with midazolam. In 2014 Feder, Charney et al. conducted a study of 41 unmedicated patients diagnosed with PTSD.[7] It was a randomised, double-blind, placebo-controlled trial with a crossover period of two weeks. They focussed on the 24-hour post-infusion response, and it showed a significant improvement for ketamine versus midazolam; this improvement persisted for some. Patients with co-morbid depressive symptoms also improved, but this did not influence ketamine's effect on PTSD. Side effects, including feelings of dissociation, were mild and transient. Three patients were given propranolol to reduce increased heart rate and blood pressure.

The authors concluded that the results of the trial required replication and extension to the use of multiple doses of ketamine. They also speculated that using ketamine for anaesthesia and pain relief for traumatic injury should be further explored as a way of preventing PTSD in these patients.

Feder et al in 2014 had shown that ketamine could be helpful in the short term for patients suffering with PTSD. Results from a further trial published in 2018 by Basant et al showed that combined mindfulness psychotherapy and ketamine is effective in treating PTSD.[18] The 20-patient study examined the length of sustained response with combined "Trauma Interventions using Mindfulness-Based Extinction and Reconsolidation" [TIMBER] and ketamine.

This was a double blind trial with a single infusion of ketamine 0.5mg/kg bodyweight given over 40 minutes combined with mindfulness-based cognitive therapy compared with a saline infusion plus the psychotherapy.

They enrolled 20 patients with moderate to severe PTSD who had been unresponsive to at least 2 medication trials and CBT over the prior 6 months.

Ketamine alone [from prior trial results] gave a 7-day response duration.

TIMBER and saline gave a 17-day response.

TIMBER and ketamine led to a 34-day response.

They also presented data suggesting that basal d-serine levels may serve as a biomarker both for the severity of PTSD symptoms and also as a predictor of clinical response.

As reported in chapter 3 Albott et al have recently examined the use of ketamine to successfully treat patients with concurrent PTSD and major depression.

Treatment of Suicidal Thinking:

[See also Chapter 8 for earlier work]

In 2016 Wei Fan et al published a study in which 42 patients with newly diagnosed cancer who presented with depression and suicidal thoughts were given a single intravenous dose of ketamine versus midazolam as the active control.[20[Patients with cancer have double the usual rate of suicide in the first 2 months following diagnosis.

Significant improvements in suicidal thinking were evident 24 and 72 hours following the ketamine infusion. By 7 days there was a numerical advantage over the midazolam group, but this did not reach clinical significance. Similarly depression scores were significantly lower at 24 hours and 72 hours post-infusion and were numerically improved at 7 days.

In 2017 Lucinda Grande described the use of repeated 1-2 hourly doses of sublingual ketamine to reduce suicidal thinking in 2 patients with a major depressive disorder who had no current intent to act on the thoughts.[21]

Ketamine was added to the their treatment regime and close outpatient follow-up was instituted.

Both were commenced on 16mg of sublingual ketamine with instructions to take repeated doses every 1-2 hours until settled.

The first man aged in his 60s described an increasing "sense of calm" after his second dose. Half an hour later he was markedly improved, smiling and joking. He was closely monitored by phone and clinic visits over the next month. He took 48 to 128 mg a day for the first two days, returned to work a week later and discontinued ketamine after a month. He continued to take an increased dose of his regular antidepressant venlafaxine.

Her second patient was diagnosed with bipolar depression and had a past history of attempted suicide. He found a dose of 8-16 mg daily over a period of 6 months was helpful in reducing suicidal thoughts when added to his medication regime together with increased support.

This was a small study but one strongly suggesting that repeated, relatively low doses of sublingual ketamine can rapidly reduce suicidal thinking, often within hours. This is in accord with my own experience that for many, but not all patients with suicidal thoughts, this can be a life-saving strategy as part of a comprehensive treatment plan.

Pierre Blier et al from Ottawa have been involved in a series of studies on the effect of intravenous ketamine [IVK] on suicidal ideation [SI] and major depression [MDD]. [22]

In a 2016 trial 19 patients with MDD and SI were given 7 IVK infusions with a midazolam control for the first infusion.

10 of the 17 completers responded to the ketamine infusions over 3 weeks with significantly lower depression scores.

Both responders and non-responders on the depression scales had lower SI scores.

They concluded that ketamine had a direct effect on lessening suicidal ideation even in patients who failed to show a reduction in depression severity with repeated infusions.

Again, in a presentation at the ENCAP congress in 2016, they described treating 27 patients, each receiving 7 intravenous ketamine infusions.

16 patients had reduced depression scores and 21 had reduced SI scores. Those whose depression scores improved had a greater reduction in SI than the non-responders, but even without reduced depression the SI scores in non-responders were both statistically significant and clinically meaningful.

In 2017 the group reported that they had now treated 34 patients of whom 50% had responded with lower depression scores. However 90% had lower SI scores once again confirming a robust effect on suicidal ideation partly independent of reductions in depression.

Wilkinson et al conducted a review of trials of intravenous ketamine in patients for whom suicidal thinking had been assessed.[23]

In this meta-analysis 10 trials, all with placebo controls, were examined. There were 167 patients out of a total of 298 who reported SI at baseline. Those given a single intravenous infusion of ketamine did better than the placebo group for up to 7 days.

Improvement in SI scores was statistically significant even when taking into account improvement in depressive symptoms. This confirmed Blier's findings that for some SI can improve even if depression scores do not. 55% of the ketamine treated patients were free of SI in 24 hours and 60% at one week.

By comparison in trials of electroconvulsive therapy [ECT] for patients with major depression and SI, 38% are free from SI after 3 treatments given in the first week and 60 % after 6 treatments given over a period of 2 weeks.

Grunebaum et al in 2018 published the results of a midazolam-controlled trial of single-dose intravenous ketamine in 80 inpatients with MDD and SI.[24]

Importantly, in this study, those with bipolar and borderline diagnoses were not excluded and 54% of the patients were currently on antidepressant medication.

At 24 hours post-infusion the response rate in the ketamine group for SI was 55% compared to 30% in the midazolam group with the difference being apparent from 2 hours post-treatment. By Cohen criteria this is a medium effect size. Interestingly, those with borderline diagnoses had the same response as those without.

Improvement on the depression scales mediated 33% of ketamine's effect on the SI scale, which was in keeping with Blier's findings.

Side effects from the treatment were short-lived and well tolerated and improvement was maintained over 6 weeks with optimised pharmacotherapy. There were 2 suicides in the ketamine group after the 6-month study period was completed.

Therefore, as the Hu and Zhang studies [see Chapter 3] have also described, combining optimized pharmacotherapy with a single dose of ketamine can have a significant effect on outcomes.

Also in 2018 Canuso et al reported on a multicentre, placebo-controlled trial of 84 inpatients with major depression and strong suicidal thoughts.[25] Patients with diagnoses of borderline personality disorder, bipolar disorder, current substance abuse and psychosis were excluded from this trial.

The group was given intranasal esketamine twice weekly for 4 weeks together with optimized pharmacotherapy. They showed significantly reduced depression scores after 4 and 24 hours post-administration and a significant improvement in SI scores after 4 hours with a numerical improvement after 24 hours. 35% of the patients had resolution of SI at 24 hours after the first dose of esketamine.

Although the dose could be reduced to 56mg, there were 5 withdrawals from the study and nausea, dizziness, dissociation, unpleasant taste and headache were the most common transient side effects.

In a review in 2018 Andrade et al concluded that there is consistent evidence that a single dose of ketamine is associated with antisuicidal benefits that can emerge within an hour of administration and persist for up to a week.[26] The improvement is in part independent of reduced depression severity. They concluded that further study is warranted.

Alcoholism and Heroin Addiction

Ketamine also has drawn interest from researchers studying alcohol addiction largely because of findings indicating that the drug's negative effects are blunted and positive effects more pronounced in people with a family history of alcoholism.

Researchers at Yale and the West Haven VA are now conducting a study to gauge the effects of ketamine on mood and alcohol consumption in patients with both depression and alcohol dependence. The theory is that there may be an underlying problem with the glutamate system in alcoholism. It may be that some—at least initially—are self-medicating depression with the use of alcohol, and as alcohol, like ketamine, acts on the NMDA receptor, they then develop tolerance and dependence.

Of course, the use of ketamine for the treatment of both alcohol and heroin addiction goes back to Krupitsky's work.

Krupitsky et al. in Russia in 2002, before regulatory changes there halted research, conducted a double-blind, randomised clinical trial comparing the relative effectiveness of high-dose (2.0 mg/kg intramuscular) to low-dose (0.2 mg/kg intramuscular) administrations of ketamine for the psychotherapeutic treatment of heroin addiction.[8] Two-year follow-up data indicated that high-dose ketamine was more effective in inducing reduced craving and higher abstinence rates as well as positive psychological changes.

In a further study, he reported that heroin-addicted patients responded better to three sessions of ketamine-assisted psychotherapy, having twice the rate of abstinence of those receiving only one.[9]

Krupitsky's colleague Kungurtsev developed a transpersonal psychological therapy as a way of trying to better utilise the profound mystical experiences some experienced with ketamine. He found that successful treatment of alcoholism with ketamine was correlated with a changed spiritual outlook in the same way that 12-step programs also achieve success by changing addicts' spiritual outlook.[10]

The combination of ketamine with psychotherapy was first studied in Argentina in 1973. There has recently been renewed interest in the use of psychedelic agents, including ketamine, in this area. In 1973, the Iranian psychiatrist E. Khorramzadeh, MD, published the first report on the use of ketamine as an adjunct to psychotherapy.[11]

His patients reported a number of different effects. Many vividly recalled painful childhood events. 'I always desired to make nasty remarks but dared not,' said one. 'The injection took away the discomfort in my chest,' reported another. 'My heavy burden of sin is gone now', 'I now feel care-free, with no worries', and 'As a child I always wanted to shout but they did not let me' were other responses. In fact, 91% of the patients were still doing well six months later.

Many of the patients treated with ketamine for depressive disorders over the last 15 years have had coexisting anxiety symptoms which have also improved. Ketamine certainly relieves anxiety in rodents.

A study in 2009 showed that ketamine given to rats gave anxiolytic-like effects without reducing general activity. In addition, ketamine produced electrical changes in the hippocampus similar to those produced by the classic anxiolytic diazepam and other medications helpful for anxiety conditions.[12]

More recently ketamine has been shown to be helpful for those experiencing alcohol-withdrawal symptoms and it is being further studied as a longer-term treatment for alcohol dependence.

Cocaine dependence:

E Dakwar et al. have been investigating whether ketamine can be helpful for people dependent on cocaine.[27] In a trial in 2017 they gave 20 non-depressed, cocaine dependent patients either a 0.71 mg/kg infusion of ketamine over 52 minutes or midazolam infused for the same time.

The patients were then asked to choose between gifts of cocaine or money.

The participants who received ketamine made on average 1.6 choices out of 5 for the cocaine option compared to 4.33 out of 5 by those who received midazolam. The reduced craving persisted for several days post-ketamine.

Overall ketamine reduced cocaine self-administration by 67% compared to midazolam at 24 hours post-infusion.

Dakwar has also combined ketamine with mindfulness training for cocaine addicts. He has reported that preliminary results from this combined treatment were very positive. At 2 weeks, 49% of those receiving ketamine had ceased using cocaine, compared with only 9% of those receiving a placebo infusion. He postulates that ketamine "quiets the mind" and gives patients about a week's window of opportunity to create new patterns of thought and behaviour.

It is thought that addictions are associated with 'rewiring' in the reward centres of the brain. Once this occurs people can have persistent cravings even if they have stopped taking the drug, suggesting that the rewiring has not altered. Given ketamine's known ability to induce both neurogenesis and synaptic change it becomes clearer why this has now been shown to be helpful in the treatment of a variety of addictions including alcohol, heroin and cocaine.

Eating Disorders

To examine in more detail the use of ketamine for the treatment of eating disorders, see the work by Mills (1998) in chapter 3, 'The History of Use of Ketamine in Depression'.[13]

Borderline Disorder.

There have been anecdotal reports appearing on online forums from people diagnosed with borderline disorder who have experienced improved mood regulation and reduced suicidal thinking after taking ketamine. Trials on the use of ketamine in patients with suicidal ideation have shown that this is reduced in patients with borderline disorder at the same level as in those with other diagnoses. A full clinical trial has recently been established to specifically examine the use of ketamine in borderline patients with suicidal thinking.

Depression with Psychosis:

Patients with a past or current diagnosis of psychosis are usually excluded from clinical trials of ketamine, as it is feared that the psychotomimetic ["psychosis-mimicking"] acute effects of ketamine may trigger or worsen their condition. Early studies in the 1990's of administering ketamine to patients with psychosis did show increased psychotic-like symptoms e.g. hallucinations, derealisation and delusional beliefs. However, these rapidly resolved and long term follow up of these patients did not reveal any persisting problems.

There have now been a number of case reports outlining success following ketamine therapy being given to patients with current psychosis and depression.

Pennybaker et al in 2017 reviewed information concerning 12 patients with a history of psychosis taken from 3 separate clinical trials and established that these patients experienced significant improvement in depressive symptoms, albeit not quite as much as those without a history of psychosis.[32]

At 40 minutes post infusion these patients had more dissociative [but not psychotomimetic] symptoms than their peers; however, the dissociative symptoms did not persist.

They concluded that physicians should not assume that a single infusion of ketamine would exacerbate psychotic symptoms in predisposed patients.

Da Frota et al in 2017 updated the progress of two patients with psychotic features complicating severe depressive episodes whom they had been treating with intravenous ketamine for over 12 months.[33]

Both were being managed with monthly maintenance ketamine without significant side effects.

They had first described these patients in 2016.[34]

The first patient was a 52 year old woman with a long history of unipolar depression with psychotic features who presented with depressive symptoms, auditory hallucinations and paranoid delusions and was reporting a suicide plan to drink antifreeze. All of these symptoms subsided rapidly after her first infusion during which she experienced headache, fatigue and mild dissociative symptoms. She was given ketamine 0.5mg/kg bodyweight over 40 minutes.

The second patient was a 55 year old woman with a long and severe psychiatric history of schizoaffective disorder who presented with depressive symptoms and severe suicidal ideation involving driving a car off the road or overdosing on pills. The patient was withdrawn, whispering, catatonic, and responding to internal stimuli. Because of severity of past depressive episodes and the fact that she had previously received ketamine as the anaesthetic agent with electroconvulsive therapy with a robust antidepressant effect to the treatment even though no seizure was induced, ketamine infusion was administered. After her first infusion dramatic improvement occurred in both her mood and psychotic symptoms.

Ayub et al in 2018 presented the results of a trial in which 4 patients with depression and psychotic symptoms were treated with esketamine, in one instance given intravenously and in the remainder subcutaneously.[35]

3 improved rapidly with single doses of esketamine with the benefits persisting for several weeks while one did not improve despite 3 more weekly treatments.

It is now clear that neither a past history of psychosis nor current psychotic symptoms are contraindications to a trial of ketamine therapy in patients suffering from depression. It would be of interest to see whether catatonic symptoms, which are often mood disorder based, also respond to ketamine.

Physical Conditions

Parkinson's Disease:

Sherman et al in 2016 described the use of ketamine to help patients who had developed dyskinesia [abnormal involuntary movements] in response to taking L-Dopa to treat their Parkinson's disease.[28]
5 patients were given 50-96 hour infusions of ketamine - a strategy often used for patients with chronic pain disorders. All showed a strong and for some a prolonged response for months following the treatment. Associated depressive symptoms also improved. They are now proceeding to a full clinical trial.

Migraines:

Lauritsen et al in 2016 described a retrospective chart review of the results of treating refractory migraine with intravenous ketamine.[29] 6 patients were given ketamine beginning at 0.1mg/kg/hour with the dose increasing hourly as tolerated. All patients responded with substantial short-term improvement in symptoms with pain scores reducing from 9/10 to below 3/10. The average infusion time was 44 hours.

Priapism:

Priapism [a persistent painful erection] is an adverse effect of medications often used to treat psychiatric disorders.[30] Patients may require surgical intervention to induce detumescence.

Park et al described a case report in which ketamine used alone was able to bring relief. Ketamine, at an anaesthetic dose of 4mg/kg bodyweight, was given intramuscularly to a 15-year-old boy in preparation for surgical drainage of the penis. However within 2 minutes the erection had subsided and surgery was deemed unnecessary. There have been other case reports dating from 1972 describing similar outcomes from ketamine therapy.

In the interest of brevity, I will list rather than detail more of the physical conditions and medical applications in which ketamine is currently being used:

1. anaesthesia (the most commonly used anaesthetic worldwide)
2. acute sedation of violent, agitated, and delirious patients
3. acute pain (used alone or in combination with opiates)
4. treatment-refractory chronic pain
5. status epilepticus
6. status asthmaticus
7. traumatic brain injury
8. stroke (being investigated)
9. Alzheimer's disease (being investigated)
10. Parkinson's disease (being investigated).

References

1. *Australian Doctor* editorial, June 2015.
2. Logan K. Wink, 'Intranasal Ketamine Treatment in an Adult with Autism Spectrum Disorder', *Journal of Clinical Psychiatry*, 75/8 (2014), 835 836. DOI:10.4088/JCP.13cr08917.
3. Christina T. Loguidice, 'Rett Syndrome Research Trust Awards $1.3 Million for Low-Dose Ketamine Phase 2 Trial', *Rare Disease Report* (04 March 2015).
4. J. E. Berner, 'Intranasal Ketamine for Intermittent Explosive Disorder: A Case Report', *Journal of Clinical Psychiatry*, 68/8 (2007), 1305.
5. Carolyn I. Rodriguez, Lawrence S. Kegeles, A. Levinson, T. Feng, S. Marcus, D. Vermes, P. Flood, HB. Simpson, 'Randomized

Controlled Crossover Trial of Ketamine in Obsessive-Compulsive Disorder: Proof-of-Concept', *Neuropsychopharmacology*, 38/12 (November 2013): 2475–2483. Published online 17 July 2013. DOI: 10.1038/npp.2013.150.

6. Govinda, Social anxiety forum.

7. Adriana Feder, Michael K. Parides, James W. Murrough, Andrew M. Perez, Julia E. Morgan, Shireen Saxena, Katherine Kirkwood, Marije aan het Rot, Kyle A. B. Lapidus, Le-Ben Wan, Dan Iosifescu, Dennis S. Charney, 'Efficacy of Intravenous Ketamine for Treatment of Chronic Posttraumatic Stress Disorder: A Randomized Clinical Trial', *JAMA Psychiatry* (16 April 2014).

8. E. Krupitsky, A. Burakov, T. Romanova, I. Dunaevsky, R. Strassman, A. Grinenko, 'Ketamine Psychotherapy for Heroin Addiction: Immediate Effects and Two-Year Follow-Up', *Journal of Substance Abuse Treatment*, 23/4 (December 2002), 273–83.

9. E. M. Krupitsky, A. M. Burakov, I. V. Dunaevsky, T. N. Romanova, T. Y. Slavina, A. Y. Grinenko, 'Single versus Repeated Sessions of Ketamine-Assisted Psychotherapy for People with Heroin Dependence', *Journal of Psychoactive Drugs* (31 March 2007).

10. I. Kungurtsev, 'Death-Rebirth Psychotherapy with Ketamine', *The Albert Hofmann Foundation Bulletin*, 2 (1991), 1–6.

11. 'Ketamine Peril and Promise', xvii/1 (spring–summer 2007).

12. 'Corrigendum to "Anxiolytic- and Antidepressant-Like Properties of Ketamine in Behavioral and Neurophysiological Animal Models" [Neuroscience 161 (2009) 359–369]', *Neuroscience*, 162/4 (15 September 2009), 1438–1439. DOI of original article: 10.1016/j.neuroscience.2009.03.038.

13. I. H. Mills, G. R. Park, A. R. Manara, R. J. Merriman, 'Treatment of compulsive behaviour in eating disorders with intermittent ketamine infusions', *QJM*, 91/7 (July 1998), 493–503.

New References:

15. Glue, P., Medlicott, N. J., Harland, S., Neehoff, S., Anderson-Fahey, B., Le Nedelec, M., . . . McNaughton, N. (2017). Ketamine's dose-related effects on anxiety symptoms in patients with treatment refractory anxiety disorders.

Journal of Psychopharmacology, 31(10), 1302-1305. doi: 10.1177/0269881117705089

16. Glue, P., Neehoff, S. M., Medlicott, N. J., Gray, A., Kibby, G., & McNaughton, N. (2018). Safety and efficacy of maintenance ketamine treatment in patients with treatment-refractory generalised anxiety and social anxiety disorders. Journal of Psychopharmacology, 32(6), 663-667. doi: 10.1177/0269881118762073

17. Taylor, J. H., Landeros-Weisenberger, A., Coughlin, C., Mulqueen, J., Johnson, J. A., Gabriel, D., . . . Bloch, M. H. (2017). Ketamine for Social Anxiety Disorder: A Randomized, Placebo-Controlled Crossover Trial. Neuropsychopharmacology, 43, 325. doi: 10.1038/npp.2017.194

18. Pradhan, B., Mitrev, L., Moaddell, R., & Wainer, I. W. (2018). d-Serine is a potential biomarker for clinical response in treatment of post-traumatic stress disorder using (R,S)-ketamine infusion and TIMBER psychotherapy: A pilot study. Biochim Biophys Acta, 1866(7), 831-839. doi: 10.1016/j.bbapap.2018.03.006

19. Singh et al Letter May 2018, JAMA.

20. Fan, W., Yang, H., Sun, Y., Zhang, J., Li, G., Zheng, Y., & Liu, Y. (2017). Ketamine rapidly relieves acute suicidal ideation in cancer patients: a randomized controlled clinical trial. Oncotarget, 8(2), 2356-2360. doi: 10.18632/oncotarget.13743

21. Grande, L. A. (2017). Sublingual Ketamine for Rapid Relief of Suicidal Ideation. Prim Care Companion CNS Disord, 19(2). doi: 10.4088/PCC.16l02012

22. Phillips, J. L., Norris, S., Talbot, J., Owoeye, O., & Blier, P. (2016). PS222. Ketamine Exerts a Prolonged Reduction in Suicidal Ideation Independent of its Antidepressant Effects. International Journal of Neuropsychopharmacology, 19(Suppl 1), 81-81. doi: 10.1093/ijnp/pyw043.222

23. Wilkinson, S. T., Ballard, E. D., Bloch, M. H., Mathew, S. J., Murrough, J. W., Feder, A., . . . Sanacora, G. (2017). The Effect of a Single Dose of Intravenous Ketamine on Suicidal Ideation: A Systematic Review and Individual Participant Data Meta-Analysis. American Journal of Psychiatry, 175(2), 150-158. doi: 10.1176/appi.ajp.2017.17040472

25. Canuso, C. M., Singh, J. B., Fedgchin, M., Alphs, L., Lane, R., Lim, P., . . . Drevets, W. C. (2018). Efficacy and Safety of Intranasal Esketamine for the Rapid Reduction of Symptoms of Depression and Suicidality in Patients at Imminent Risk for Suicide: Results of a Double-Blind, Randomized, Placebo-Controlled Study. American Journal of Psychiatry, 175(7), 620-630. doi: 10.1176/appi.ajp.2018.17060720

26. Andrade, C. (2018). Ketamine for Depression, 6: Effects on Suicidal Ideation and Possible Use as Crisis Intervention in Patients at Suicide Risk. J Clin Psychiatry, 79(2). doi: 10.4088/JCP.18f12242

27. Dakwar, E., Hart, C. L., Levin, F. R., Nunes, E. V., & Foltin, R. W. (2017). Cocaine self-administration disrupted by the N-methyl-D-aspartate receptor antagonist ketamine: a randomized, crossover trial. Mol Psychiatry, 22(1), 76-81. doi: 10.1038/mp.2016.39

28. Sherman, S. J., Estevez, M., Magill, A. B., & Falk, T. (2016). Case Reports Showing a Long-Term Effect of Subanesthetic Ketamine Infusion in Reducing l-DOPA-Induced Dyskinesias. Case Rep Neurol, 8(1), 53-58. doi: 10.1159/000444278

29. Lauritsen, C., Mazuera, S., Lipton, R. B., & Ashina, S. (2016). Intravenous ketamine for subacute treatment of refractory chronic migraine: a case series. J Headache Pain, 17(1), 106. doi: 10.1186/s10194-016-0700-3

30. Park, D. B., & Hayden, G. E. (2015). Ketamine Saves the Day: Priapism in a Pediatric Psychiatric Patient. Pediatr Emerg Care, 31(7), 508-510. doi: 10.1097/pec.0000000000000485

32. Pennybaker, S. J., Luckenbaugh, D. A., Park, L. T., Marquardt, C. A., & Zarate, C. A., Jr. (2017). Ketamine and Psychosis History: Antidepressant Efficacy and Psychotomimetic Effects Postinfusion. Biol Psychiatry, 82(5), e35-e36. doi: 10.1016/j.biopsych.2016.08.041

33. Da Frota Ribeiro, C. M et al. (2017). Update on Long-Term Effects of Ketamine in Two Patients with Depression in the Context of Psychotic Symptoms. DOI:http://dx.doi.org/10.1016/j.biopsych.2017.01.012

34. Da Frota Ribeiro, C. M., Sanacora, G., Hoffman, R., & Ostroff, R. (2016). The Use of Ketamine for the Treatment of Depression

in the Context of Psychotic Symptoms. Biological Psychiatry, 79(9), e65-e66. doi: 10.1016/j.biopsych.2015.05.016

35. Ajub, E., & Lacerda, A. L. T. (2018). Efficacy of Esketamine in the Treatment of Depression With Psychotic Features: A Case Series. Biological Psychiatry, 83(1), e15-e16. doi: 10.1016/j.biopsych.2017.06.011

Chapter 10

Research into Racemic Ketamine Derivatives and Analogues

What are the alternatives to ketamine for the treatment of depressive illness that are currently exciting researchers? Most of the following agents are still being investigated, but there are a few that are currently available to patients.

First, let us examine the components of racemic ketamine, the mixture used by most doctors worldwide. It is made from a combination of R- and S-ketamine (arketamine and esketamine), both of which have antidepressant effects.

Arketamine

Arketamine is the $R(-)$ enantiomer (mirror image) of ketamine. It is considered to be less potent than esketamine in anaesthetic, analgesic, and sedative effects, but it has not yet been approved or marketed in its own right. By contrast, arketamine shows greater, longer-lasting, and rapid antidepressant effects in animal models of depression compared to esketamine, and it has been suggested that this difference may have been due to the different activity of both arketamine and esketamine and their respective metabolites at the $\langle_7$-nicotinic receptor.

Interestingly, there do not appear to be plans at present to trial arketamine as a treatment in its own right.

Esketamine

Janssen, a subsidiary of the pharmaceutical company Johnson and Johnson, is developing the S-isomer of ketamine [esketamine] as an intranasal formulation.

They have been working towards a US Food and Drug Administration [FDA] approval for esketamine, both for use in treatment-resistant depression and for depressed patients at imminent risk of suicide.

On September the 4th 2018 Janssen announced that they had submitted a new drug application to the FDA for esketamine nasal spray to be used for treatment-resistant depression in adults.

They plan to submit a marketing authorisation application to the European Medicines Agency (EMA) for the esketamine treatment-resistant depression indication later in 2018. They stated that "Esketamine nasal spray will be self-administered by patients under the supervision of health care professionals."

By mid 2018 Janssen had conducted five pivotal Phase 3 studies of esketamine nasal spray in patients with treatment-resistant depression. These clinical studies included three short-term randomised, double blind, active-controlled studies (fixed dose, flexible dose and a flexible dose study in patients $\geq$ 65 years), one double blind, randomised, maintenance of effect study and one open-label, long-term safety study. The results from these studies were then presented to the FDA as regulatory filings for esketamine nasal spray in treatment-resistant depression.

These phase 3 studies defined 'treatment-resistant' as patients who had not responded to two or more conventional antidepressants given in adequate dose and duration for the current episode of depression.

Daly, Singh et al presented the results of Janssen's Phase 2 study of intranasal esketamine for treatment-resistant depression [TRD] in the December 2017 edition of JAMA Psychiatry.[8] They examined 67 patients with TRD who had previously failed two adequate courses of antidepressants either in the current episode or over 2 episodes of illness.

Intranasal ketamine was added to their current medications at doses of 28, 56, and 84 mg and a further group received placebo, the doses being given twice weekly.

After one week the non-responders in the placebo group were randomised to all four options.

After two weeks all those who agreed entered an open-phase starting at 56mg with dose adjustments made thereafter according to side effects and responses.

They took ketamine twice weekly for 2 weeks, thereafter the dose was taken weekly for 3 weeks, then every 2 weeks for 4 weeks and then stopped with a further 4 weeks of monitoring done off ketamine.

Four patients discontinued treatment [all in the active treatment group] due to syncope, headache, dissociation and ectopic pregnancy.

Overall, the higher the dose the more side effects, albeit transitory.

Response rates were 38%, 36%, 50%, 10% - [corresponding to the 28mg, 56mg, 84mg and placebo groups]

Remission rates were 13%, 27%, 40%, 10% - [corresponding to the 28mg, 56mg, 84mg and placebo groups]

These rapid and significant improvements were sustained over two months at decreasing dose intervals. A clear dose-response effect was apparent for both benefit and side effects.

Janssen has also presented a study on patients with suicidal thinking and major depression [see Chapter 9, Canuso et al.]

In May 2018 Janssen presented results from a trial involving 223 patients from 39 multinational centres. This was a randomised, double blind trial with a placebo control using flexible dosing of intranasal ketamine.

Patients had been diagnosed with moderate to severe major depressive disorder and had failed 2 antidepressant medications in their current illness episode. They were given either 56mg or 84 mg of intranasal ketamine [INK] twice weekly together with a newly initiated antidepressant or a placebo spray along with a newly initiated antidepressant.

Primary efficacy end point measurements on the Madras depression scale from baseline to 28 days showed statistically significant improvements.

Response rates in the esketamine group were 69% versus 52% in the control group and remission rates were 52% in the esketamine group compared to 30% in the control group. Side effects reported by more than 10% of patients included short-term metallic taste, vertigo, dizziness, headaches, dissociation and most frequently nausea and vertigo. [26%].

Interestingly, there was a higher than usual response rate in the placebo group perhaps reflecting the extra support received during clinical trials and better compliance with treatment.

For the esketamine arm there was an average 4-point reduction in the Madras depression rating scale. To put this into context typical antidepressant trials usually obtain a 2-3 point drop in the Madras and reductions above 1.9 can be clinically meaningful.

Janssen has also presented the results of a study in elderly [65 and above] patients with treatment-resistant depression. This was a multicentre study involving 138 patients in which a newly initiated antidepressant was added to both the esketamine and placebo arms.

The primary endpoint of a 4.0-drop in the Madras after 28 days was just missed [3.6]. However, when the subgroup of those over 75 years was removed statistical significance was attained.

Overall response rates were 27% versus 13% in the control group with remission rates of 17% versus 7% in the control group.

Findings on safety were similar to previous studies in younger populations.

A further report by Janssen presented in 2018 was a long-term study into relapse prevention.[9]

705 patients were examined in this phase 3 trial which involved patients who had previously responded and were stable after 4 months treatment with intranasal esketamine and a newly initiated antidepressant.

This further trial compared ongoing treatment with either esketamine and the previously initiated antidepressant or a placebo nasal spray and the previously initiated antidepressant

The overall findings were both clinically meaningful and statistically significant.

Overall the esketamine group who were stable "remitters" had a 51% reduced risk of relapse compared to the placebo group. Those who were stable "responders" had a 70% reduced risk of relapse.

Of those in stable remission 26% of the esketamine group relapsed compared to 45% in the placebo group. Of the stable responders 26% in the esketamine group relapsed compared to 58% in the placebo arm.

Maintenance ketamine therapy was shown to be safe and tolerable as in the previous studies. 6 patients experienced adverse events that were considered to be possibly or probably ketamine-related.

This trial clearly demonstrates that long-term maintenance therapy with intranasal ketamine does indeed reduce the risk of relapse; this is in accord with other maintenance trials using racemic ketamine.

Janssen's next trial explored the long-term safety of administering intranasal esketamine. They assessed 802 patients who had been treated for one year.

This was a phase 3 open label trial in which patients who had previously taken doses of intranasal ketamine varying between 28, 56 and 84mg intermittently for 16 weeks were enrolled and followed for 12 months.

Over the 12 month period the short-term side effects experienced by more than 10% of patients were:

Dizziness 32%
Dissociation 27%
Nausea 25%
Headache 25%
Drowsiness 17%
Metallic taste 12%
Hypoalgesia [numbing] 12%
Vertigo 11%
Vomiting 11%

There were no reported laboratory test abnormalities. This is an important finding as long-term, high dose recreational use has been associated with bladder and liver problems. There were no reports of ketamine misuse.

55 of the 802 patients reported 68 treatment emergent side effects in total. Of these 4 patients had effects "probably" related to esketamine [depression, delirium, anxiety and delusion, suicidal ideation and a suicide attempt].

Although this study was not designed to measure efficacy, taking intranasal esketamine appeared to sustain improvements in depressive symptoms over the 12 month period with little change in the overall response and remission rates over that time.

In summary, clinically meaningful and statistically significant improvement has been demonstrated using the strategy of adding intranasal ketamine to newly initiated antidepressants. Long term safety over 12 months of treatment has been established and this is in accord with the data presented by Feifel et al for 7544 patients taking parenteral racemic ketamine over prolonged periods of time. [see Chapter 6]

It is very interesting that Janssen has adopted the strategy of Hu and Zhang [See Chapter 3] of combining esketamine with antidepressant therapy rather than treating patients with esketamine alone. Perhaps they see this as an approach more likely to win favour with the FDA.

Whatever the reasons, they have presented very important data illustrating the safety and efficacy of the long-term use of esketamine in large numbers of patients in multiple centres, thus confirming what other prescribers administering racemic ketamine have been reporting in recent years.

Next there are the breakdown products that appear in the body as ketamine is metabolised by the liver—norketamine and hydroxynorketamine.

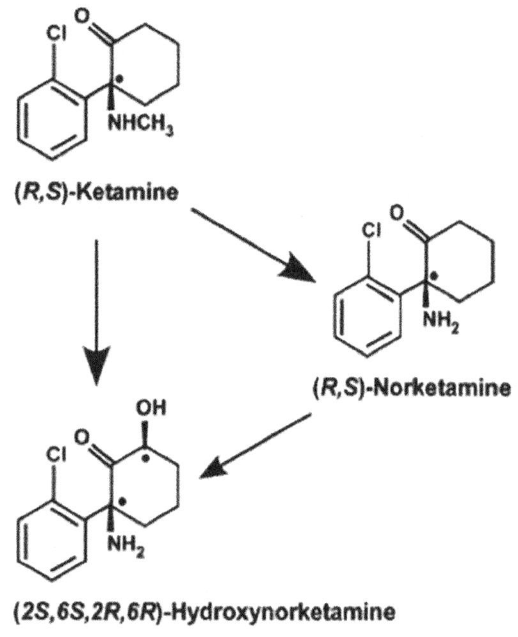

(R,S)-Ketamine

(R,S)-Norketamine

(2S,6S,2R,6R)-Hydroxynorketamine

Image courtesy of Anaesthesiology 2104, 121: 149-59

Norketamine

Norketamine is the major active metabolite of ketamine. Like ketamine, norketamine acts on the NMDA receptor but is weaker as an anaesthetic. Compared to ketamine, norketamine is a stronger antagonist of the ζ_7-nicotinic acetylcholine receptor and produces rapid antidepressant effects in animal models which correlate with its activity at this receptor.

I am not aware of any studies specifically targeting the use of norketamine, but there is great interest in the next link in the metabolic chain, hydroxynorketamine (HNK).

Hydroxynorketamine

Irving Wainer (senior investigator with the Intramural Research Program at the National Institute on Aging, Baltimore) said that they had found that the HNK compound significantly contributes to the antidepressive effects of ketamine in animals but doesn't produce the same degree of sedation or anaesthesia as ketamine, thus making HNK an attractive alternative as an antidepressant in humans.

They gave rats intravenous doses of ketamine, HNK, and norketamine. The effect each had on stimulating certain cellular pathways of the rats' brains was examined after 20, 30, and 60 minutes. They used brain tissue from drug-free rats as the control.

They discovered that HNK, like ketamine, not only produced potent and rapid antidepressant effects but also stimulated neuroregenerative pathways and initiated the regrowth of neurons in rats' brains. HNK also appeared to have several advantages over ketamine in that it was 1,000 times more potent, did not act as an anaesthetic agent, and potentially could be given orally.

They also found that HNK reduced the production of D-serine, a chemical found in the body, overproduction of which is associated with neurodegenerative disorders, such as Alzheimer's and Parkinson's diseases. This raises the tantalising prospect that HNK could be helpful in a range of neurodegenerative disorders.[1]

Ketamine Analogues

Next, there are those compounds that work in similar fashion to ketamine, acting on the NMDA receptor, the ketamine analogues.

Researchers such as Carlos Zarate from the NIMH consider that there is not yet enough evidence available for them to seek approval from the FDA to use ketamine for the treatment of depression. Such approval would lead to medical insurers covering this in their policies, thus reducing the high costs charged to patients in the USA. Interestingly, some insurers cover ketamine infusions for pain, which is also an off-label use.

However, some researchers and pharmaceutical companies think the future may lie in more selective ketamine analogues that work at the same receptors but lack some of the dissociative side effects that occur in treatments with higher doses of intravenous ketamine.

GLYX-13

The pharmaceutical company Naurex is working on GLYX-13 (rapastinel), a novel NMDA receptor glycine-site functional partial agonist, which has shown success in phase 2 trials. It has been reported to have antidepressant effects within 24 hours, which lasted up to 7 days in MDD patients who had failed one or more antidepressant medications. There were no dissociative effects.

It is conceivable that rapastinel, now under development by Allergan, could come to market in 2020 or 2021. It is now in phase 3 clinical trials for treating both treatment-resistant depression and acute suicidal crisis associated with depression.

In a small, preliminary clinical study rapastinel rapidly reduced symptoms of OCD, although the effect was not long lasting. The drug was well tolerated, causing none of the dissociative side effects associated with ketamine.

NRX-1074

NRX-1074 is an orally bioavailable, selective partial agonist of the glycine site of the NMDA receptor. This is another drug being developed by Naurex for the treatment of major depressive disorder, and its mechanism of action and effects are similar to those of rapastinel (GLYX-13). However, NRX-1074 is said to be several thousand times more potent by weight and, unlike GLYX-13, is orally active. NRX-1074 has shown rapid antidepressant effects in preclinical models of depression, is well tolerated, and lacks the dissociative effects of other NMDA receptor antagonists, such as ketamine. NRX 1074, now known as apimostinel, has completed phase 2 trials

CERC-301

CERC-301 is an orally active, selective NMDA receptor subunit 2B (NR2B) antagonist that is under development by Cerecor as a therapy for treatment-resistant depression. In November 2013, phase 2 clinical trials were initiated, and in the same month, CERC-301 received the 'fast track' designation from the Food and Drug Administration for treatment-resistant depression. A pilot study was published in 2012, and a phase 2 trial was completed in 2014.

In November 2016 came the following announcement "Cerecor's Phase II clinical trial of CERC-301 to treat MDD fails to meet primary endpoint."

AV-101

AV-101 is an orally active agent that produces a glycine binding site NMDA receptor antagonist. AV-101 is in clinical development by VistaGen Therapeutics, Inc. as a potential new-generation, fast-acting antidepressant as well as for other central nervous system indications. The initial phase 2 clinical study of AV-101 began in 2015 and was focused on treatment-resistant depression (TRD).

However, other companies developing analogues of ketamine have not been as successful. Roche's development of the drug decoglurant, which targets the glutamate system, was terminated due to a lack of efficacy. AstraZeneca's development of lanicemine, an NMDA channel blocker, has also been halted.

Other currently available agents which have shown preliminary evidence of efficacy for the treatment of depressive disorders include scopolamine,[2] sarcosine,[3] nitrous oxide,[4] D-cycloserine,[5,6] and botox.[7]

The growing interest in the mechanisms of ketamine's actions in the treatment of depression has led to a new focus on the glutamate system and its contribution to psychiatric disorder. In addition, pharmaceutical companies who had largely withdrawn from research in psychiatry have now returned with the tantalising prospect of discovering new patentable compounds.

References

1. Jolynn Tumolo, 'Ketamine By-Product Shows Promise for Treating Depression without Side Effects', Psych Congress Network 2015.

2. C. Han, C. U. Pae, 'Oral Scopolamine Augmentation for Major Depression', *Expert Review Neurotherapeutics*, 13/1 (January 2013), 19–21. DOI: 10.1586/ern.12.150.

3. Chih-Chia Huang, I-Hua Wei, Chieh-Liang Huang, Kuang-Ti Chen, Mang-Hung Tsai, Priscilla Tsai, Rene Tun, Kuo-Hao Huang, Yue-Cune Chang, Hsien-Yuan Lane, Guochuan Emil Tsai, 'Inhibition of Glycin Transporter-I as a Novel Mechanism for the Treatment of Depression', *Biological Psychiatry*, 74/10 (2013), 734. DOI: 10.1016/j.biopsych.2013.02.020.

4. Peter Nagele, Andreas Duma, Michael Kopec, Marie Anne Gebara, Alireza Parsoei, Marie Walker, Alvin Janski, Vassilis N. Panagopoulos, Pilar Cristancho, J. Philip Miller, Charles F. Zorumski, and Charles R. Conway. 'Nitrous Oxide for Treatment-Resistant Major Depression: A Proof-of-Concept Trial'.

5. Matthew Herper, 'Hope and Hype for New Type of Antidepressant', Pharma & Healthcare (24 June 2015).

6. Cheri A. Levinson, Thomas L. Rodebaugh, Laura Fewell, Andrea E. Kass, Elizabeth N. Riley, Lynn Stark, Kimberly McCallum, and Eric J. Lenze, *Journal of Clinical Psychiatry*, 76/6 (2015), e787–e793. DOI: 10.4088/JCP.14m09299.

7. Matthew Herper, 'Botox Seems To Ease Depression', Pharma & Healthcare (20 May 2015).

8. Daly, E. J., Singh, J. B., Fedgchin, M., Cooper, K., Lim, P., Shelton, R. C., . . . Drevets, W. C. (2018). Efficacy and Safety of Intranasal Esketamine Adjunctive to Oral Antidepressant Therapy in Treatment-Resistant Depression: A Randomized Clinical Trial. JAMA Psychiatry, 75(2), 139-148. doi: 10.1001/jamapsychiatry.2017.3739

9. John Carroll J&J racks up a fresh set of positive pivotal data for depression drug esketamine — but questions linger on safety. May 31, 2018 01:49 PM EDT – Endpoint news

Chapter 11

Why Is It Taking So Long?

The first trial showing ketamine to be an effective, rapidly acting treatment for depression was published in 2000. How can it be that 15 years on there is still division and uncertainty about its use?

The Ketamine Advocacy Network has some opinions. Dennis Hartman, who continues to be helped by prescribed ketamine, established the network in 2012. The website explains:

> The Ketamine Advocacy Network was founded at the National Institutes of Health in 2012 by ketamine clinical trial volunteers. They personally experienced the power ketamine has to rapidly relieve the excruciating pain of refractory depression.
>
> The founders quickly learned how difficult it is to get ongoing ketamine therapy from local doctors at affordable rates. And they encountered firsthand the powerful forces preventing widespread adoption of the treatment. The Ketamine Advocacy Network was born from their desire to overcome these obstacles and share the relief they experienced with fellow sufferers.
>
> Since 2012, our ranks have grown to include alumnae from other clinical studies, patients of ketamine clinics, doctors and administrators who run those clinics, and concerned loved ones. We all share the same desire to spread

awareness and acceptance of this powerful new weapon against depression, bipolar, and PTSD.[1]

I would recommend going to the website which has a wealth of ketamine-related information available as well as discussion forums: www.ketamineadvocacynetwork.org.

The network describes three main factors that they see as having impeded both the progress of research and access to ketamine treatment.

1. opposition from pharmaceutical companies
2. opposition from psychiatrists
3. opposition from researchers.

As far as the pharmaceutical companies are concerned, because ketamine has long been out of patent, they have no financial incentive to fund further research. Such research is extremely expensive, and given that any other company can use the results to promote their cheap generic version, it just does not make sense for them to proceed.

Instead they are devoting their efforts to subtly 'tweaking' ketamine to find something patentable, e.g. by giving it intranasally or looking for compounds that work in a similar fashion to ketamine. If they are successful, these 'new' treatments will make huge profits for their developers. The major flaw with this approach is that there will be no knowledge as to possible long-term harms from these new compounds, a concern that is commonly raised with ketamine now.

Psychiatrists, like any other branch of the medical profession, are conservative people. Anyone with some years of experience has seen many so-called wonder drugs appear, flame, and extinguish. Indeed, one well-known clinical maxim is that 'you should use a new treatment while it still works'. One of the big problems for the profession is that we are used to getting information about new products spoon-fed to us by their makers. So seminars, articles, and reminders are scheduled with little effort being required on our part. Given that this will not occur with ketamine, we have to find the time to do our own investigations and reach our own conclusions.

The researchers in the field usually finish their papers with the statement that 'more research is required to establish the long-term safety of using ketamine'. Given the lack of funds, these trials will rarely happen under the current free-market system, although Janssen's recent work on intranasal esketamine is giving us some clarity. Fortunately, we have canaries in the ketamine mines, those unfortunate addicts who have shown the consequences of high-dose, long-term intake. In addition, we can benefit from the experience of pain patients who have been treated with repeated infusions of ketamine over the years and also some who have been given daily sublingual ketamine for years on end.[2]

Other researchers point out that the relief is temporary, side effects can be distressing, and possible misuse of prescribed ketamine could be disastrous for the whole field. However, there is now increasing information about ways of extending the initial benefits obtained from ketamine treatment; new lower-dose strategies can minimise side effects, and taking ketamine intranasally, orally, and sublingually can significantly improve access to treatment and also reduce the costs.

Regarding abuse and addiction as a risk from treatment, it is worth pointing out that, over the past 50 years, this has very rarely been reported as a consequence of properly supervised medical treatment with ketamine.

If you want to know why Dennis Hartman feels strongly about ketamine, just read the following account:[3]

> Another of Dr Brooks' patients is Dennis Hartman. He had suffered from major refractory depressive disorder his entire life, associated with post-traumatic stress disorder, which was the result of a childhood of abuse.
>
> 'It's acute misery. Living with my depression feels like pain,' he says. 'It's something you can't show to someone, point to an injury or a wound, but it feels very much like physical pain.'
>
> 'I was aware I had a problem by the time I was in 7th grade. I had a very traumatic childhood and spent it in a state of intense fear. By the time I reached adolescence I had a pretty good idea that I wasn't able to do things like other kids were able to do.
>
> 'It felt like it was literally a character that I was talking off and hanging in the closet at the end of the day. The character looked happy, and successful, and put together, and confident, but it was being powered by a depressive sufferer who was wracked with anxiety.'

Mr Hartman spent decades working through a roster of medical and therapeutic treatments for depression.

> 'I tried every known depressive therapy, everything that doctors commonly prescribe: SSRIs, SNRIs, tricyclics, benzodiazepines. A lot of my energy in life has been spent trying to find a way to get relief from this pain.'
>
> 'On my worst days, I lost the energy. I didn't have the ability or the strength to inhabit that character any more . . . I just didn't see any way around it.'
>
> In his mid forties, Hartman decided to end his life.
>
> 'The way I thought about it in my own mind is, "It's the humane, reasonable thing to do, to end my life". There's only so much untreatable suffering that one person can be expected to endure, in their lifetime.'

He picked a date several months away in order to get his affairs in order and to avoid causing his nephew trauma during finals. While he was waiting for his date, he heard of an experimental trial using ketamine to treat depression and PTSD. He applied and was immediately accepted.

> 'The day I received my infusion my symptoms were raging. It was relatively bad—the anxiety, the anhedonia (the inability to experience pleasure), the insomnia.
>
> 'They turned on the drip and I was in a dreamlike state, like a spectator watching my thoughts unfold in front of me. Within 15 to 20 minutes of the end of the infusion, I was aware that something was different. They started to ask me questions to monitor my mood, and I had trouble pinpointing my symptoms so I could describe them.
>
> 'Within a couple of hours of the infusion I had a clear awareness that there was something missing. It didn't strike me as a wave of massive relief. It didn't feel like something was added to be, like I had superpowers. I didn't have euphoria. It was a gradual realisation over a few hours that something was missing. And what was missing was something horrible.'

'The biggest changes for me occurred within 24 hours of my first infusion. If you suffer from lifelong depression as I have, and it's all you've ever known, it becomes part of your identity. You just feel that the world is all about pain. And when I got relief from my first infusion, it was like being emancipated.'

Since discovering this treatment, Dennis has become a tireless advocate, establishing and running the Ketamine Advocacy Network, which aims to spread awareness of the treatment and connect potential patients with doctors who provide it. As of 2018 there are now more than 250 clinics and 1,000 practitioners in the US offering ketamine therapy.

References

1. Ketamine Advocacy Network. <www.ketamineadvocacynetwork.org>.
2. V. K. Jaitly, 'Sublingual Ketamine in Chronic Pain: Service Evaluation by Examining More Than 200 Patient Years of Data', *Journal of Observational Pain Medicine*, 1/2 (2013).
3. Maggie Palmer, 'Ketamine: Can This Party Drug Cure Severe Depression Overnight?', Channel SBS Two (6 April 2015).

Chapter 12

Fourteen Reasons for Doctors to Prescribe

1. It works. There are now many published and unpublished studies from around the world examining the use of ketamine for treatment-resistant depressive disorders which have reported positive results in both the short and the long term. Average response rates are approximately 70%, and remission rates are 30–50%. The response rates for the less chronic conditions are higher (De Gioannis, personal communication).

2. The short-term risks are well known and are easy to monitor and manage. We have over 50 years of experience with ketamine to inform us.

3. The long-term risks, thanks to our colleagues in pain medicine, are also known. The experiences of addicts taking regular high doses of ketamine (up to 100 times the usual treatment doses) have shown us what to be wary about.

4. Addiction is not a major hazard for those taking ketamine for medical reasons. Reports from pain physicians and psychiatrists using both ongoing parenteral and sublingual ketamine indicate rates of possible misuse at being less than one for every 200 patients treated.

5. It is affordable, particularly when the very-low-dose approach in home settings is used.

6. There is no need to withdraw patients from their current treatments before starting. Ketamine can be safely added to most medications, and it enhances psychological therapies.

7. Once people have recovered from an episode of depression, they can often reduce or stop previously partly effective treatments, easing the burden from both the side effects and the expense.

8. Ketamine, as with all other current psychiatric treatments, is not a cure, but relapses do seem to respond quickly to further administration of ketamine. There is little evidence of tolerance to the antidepressant effect.

9. Your patients will thank you at the very least for giving them the opportunity to try a new treatment. 'It gives me hope that eventually something will help' (my patient, GH).

10. It certainly beats the alternative of ongoing suffering for large numbers of people.

11. And it beats as well as the other alternative of patients self-medicating with random-quality illicit ketamine with all the attendant risks.

12. It fulfils the spirit of your Hippocratic oath—to cure sometimes, to relieve often, and to comfort always.

13. It lifts the gross national happiness index, bringing more personal joy, better relationships, and better work capability. 'I've never laughed as much as I have these past six weeks' (my patient, CR).

14. Because you can. Although Ketamine does not have an FDA-approved indication for treating depression, it is perfectly legal for doctors to prescribe it for this purpose, provided this is explained properly to the patient. Around 20% of medications currently used in psychiatry are used off label.

My 14 personal reasons for prescribing ketamine are the 14 patients of mine who have trialled this medication. Yes, they experienced very different outcomes, but they all showed the same appreciation for the chance to see if it could improve their well-being.

Some Reasons Doctors Give for Not Prescribing Ketamine

1. 'Not enough is known. We need more studies.'

   You need to read this book, do your own research, and talk to the doctors and patients using it. Unless esketamine is FDA-approved there will be no free seminars, no charming drug reps visiting, not even a pen inscribed with 'Ketamine' to remind you. There will be no other ways of finding out.

2. 'I'm not set up to monitor the initial treatment.'

   When using the very-low-dose sublingual method, taking the pulse will suffice. Ketamine is given while conducting your normal consultation. Recording blood pressure is a useful but not essential addition.

3. 'I'm worried about the medico-legal issues, the potential for abuse.'

   It's legal. See the appendix for advice about the process involved, patient information sheets, and sample consent forms. Ethically speaking, I think we would be far more likely to get into trouble for not prescribing a potentially life-saving therapy. Ketamine misuse very rarely occurs following the medical use of ketamine.

4. 'I have my own way of doing things. I don't need others to tell me what's right or wrong for me.'

   If you have a 100% success rate with your treatment, then please let us all know how you do it. If you don't, then continuing to repeat the same actions in the hope of a different outcome is not insanity—it's stupidity.

5. 'I'll refer to a ketamine clinic as I do for ECT. Let the experts do it.'

   This would be an appropriate response for some patients, particularly the acutely suicidal without sufficient support, but the vast majority of patients can be managed in your own practice with small adjustments to your skill set.

6. 'I'll wait for the full-scale, multicentre, randomised, double-blind, placebo-controlled trials—the gold standards for assessing the efficacy of psychiatric treatments.'

   Well, you'll be waiting a long time—as in forever. Although there are currently more than 600 trials planned or under way using ketamine in a variety of disorders in the USA alone, they are mostly small in scale. There is no money, no big pharmaceutical companies pushing this; it's long out of patent. These companies are working frantically to develop alternatives that are patentable and, if successful, will no doubt be very expensive for patients and taxpayers alike. But there's no guarantee they'll work as well as ketamine, nor will there be knowledge of possible long-term side effects.

If, after absorbing the contents of this book and exploring all other available information, you remain a conscientious objector to its use, then by all means refer your patient on and be sure to follow their progress with great interest.

And remember, not taking a risk is also a risk.

Chapter 13

How to Approach Your Doctor to Discuss a Trial Of Ketamine

First, for all concerned, never lose your sense of humour.

The Dos and Don'ts

We doctors like to help people, but while we understand that you're feeling low, worthless, helpless, and hopeless, we're human too, and we can at times be tired, hungry, irritable, and stressed. So please observe the following:

- Do prepare. Be calm. Carry this book.
- Don't tell us that we're uninformed dinosaurs, relics from the 'Cuckoo's Nest.'
- Do try to maintain a reasoned approach. If that's too hard in your current state of mind, bring a friend or family member for support. This can have the added benefit of giving us another view of your current condition.
- Telling us that we are lazy or incompetent for not immediately agreeing to your request may give you some short-term satisfaction but will not help towards your ultimate goal. (One contributor to the online Bluelight forum on being congratulated for finding a doctor amenable to prescribing ketamine said,

'Thanks, guys, but you have no idea how many frogs I had to kiss before finding this prince!')

- Do ask us, 'If you had a serious illness and other treatments had failed, would you be looking to try any available alternative?'
- Do explore all the alternative options. Ketamine helps around 70% of those not helped by standard treatments, so you do need a plan B.
- Be persistent. Be the squeaky door. Nag us gently.
- Give us time to think, to research, and lend us your copy of this book.
- Remind us that 'First, do no harm' does not mean 'Do nothing'.
- If all else fails, ask for a second opinion.

Chapter 14

The Future
(and the Elephants in the Room)

Through the Prospectoscope dimly

Although the most likely future scenario is that we will see incremental changes in the use of ketamine for the treatment of psychiatric disorders, there are tantalising glimpses of evidence that could lead to quantum leaps in its application.

In our current state of knowledge, the question is not whether ketamine works for treatment-resistant depression, but how can we use it most efficiently and safely?

As more doctors and patients become aware that the oral, sublingual, and intranasal administration routes are both practical and effective, the injection approaches will become a second-line therapy provided for patients either unresponsive to the simpler low-dose methods or requiring urgent therapy (e.g. those at a high risk of suicide).

For severely ill patients needing hospital care and ECT, ketamine could provide an faster-acting alternative treatment with fewer cognitive side effects. For this group of patients, it would be worth considering Correll's method of a continuous ketamine infusion, this being the approach currently being used for the more-severe pain conditions.

For many patients, a depressive illness is a chronic relapsing condition. The first episode often has a clear environmental trigger, but thereafter, the amount of stress required to cause a relapse seems to decrease. In bipolar depression, those with untreated or partly treated episodes progress particularly poorly, with their bouts of illness becoming more severe and closer together over time. This suggests that for some, perhaps those with family histories of mood disorders, we should be thinking of treating early and aggressively to try to prevent a deteriorating course.

There is mounting evidence that people who experience recurrent depressive episodes have brain shrinkage in the form of smaller hippocampal volume, which is caused by loss of connections between nerve cells rather than the death of neurones. In the early stages of illness, these losses are reversible, and treatment with ketamine rapidly increases the number and quality of these connections. It appears that the brain's capacity to heal diminishes with repeated bouts of illness.

Given this, there may be even greater value in using ketamine earlier in the disease process rather than limiting its use to treatment-resistant conditions. By administering it either alone or in combination with other therapies, we may be able limit permanent damage and promote the maximum possible healing. Thus, for certain people with higher-risk profiles, ketamine would be a first-line treatment.

Yet again our colleagues in pain medicine can show us the way. In pain management, there is now great emphasis on treating acute pain quickly and thoroughly to avoid the 'wind-up' and 'noisy brain' phenomena, which lead to the ongoing suffering and disability experienced by those in chronic pain.

As some of the side effects of the most commonly used antidepressants, the SSRIs—notably, sleep disturbance, increased weight, sexual dysfunction, and cognitive 'dulling'—can lead to patients either under-dosing or discontinuing their treatment, it is good news that ketamine does not have the same side effect profile. This means that it may be used either alone to help those who have problems with these side effects, or in combination with lower doses of the current antidepressants, thus making them more tolerable. Similarly, by enhancing the efficacy of psychotherapy, ketamine may be able to reduce the time and expense involved with this treatment.

There are also huge potential benefits in the field of palliative care. Ketamine has been shown to be effective in reducing anxiety, depression, and pain in this population without troublesome side effects.

Another field in which there is the potential for the widespread use of ketamine is the management of suicidality, where the rapid improvements in mood and the reduction of suicidal thoughts that occur with ketamine treatment would enable more resources to be directed into comprehensive treatment plans.

A major challenge for better treating depression is how to improve access to effective treatment. Over 50% of people who suffer from depressive illnesses do not seek care partly because of perceived stigma and partly due to the belief that our current treatments do more harm than good. The big problem with this is that although in milder and first episodes there is a natural improvement over time, this on average takes nine months, and people can be left with residual low-level symptoms, which leaves them more vulnerable to further episodes and a deteriorating course.

Consequently, the holy grail of depression treatment is to find an approach that works quickly to reduce suffering, has tolerable side effects, is both practical and affordable, and causes the least disruption to people's lives. It is here that the use of low-dose sublingual ketamine shows so much potential.

And now to a quantum leap:

Background

Stress exposure is one of the greatest risk factors for psychiatric illnesses like major depressive disorder and post-traumatic stress disorder. However, not all individuals exposed to stress develop affective disorders. Stress resilience, the ability to experience stress without developing persistent psychopathology, varies from individual to individual. Enhancing stress resilience in at-risk populations could potentially protect against stress-induced psychiatric disorders. Despite this fact, no resilience-enhancing pharmaceuticals have been identified.

Methods

Using a chronic social defeat (SD) stress model, learned helplessness (LH), and a chronic corticosterone (CORT) model in mice, we tested if ketamine could protect against depressive-like behaviour. Mice were administered a single dose of saline or ketamine and then 1 week later were subjected to 2 weeks of SD, LH training, or 3 weeks of CORT.

Results:

SD robustly and reliably induced depressive-like behaviour in control mice. Mice treated with prophylactic ketamine were protected against the deleterious effects of SD in the forced swim test and in the dominant interaction test. We confirmed these effects in LH and the CORT model. In the LH model, latency to escape was increased following training, and this effect was prevented by ketamine. In the CORT model, a single dose of ketamine blocked stress-induced behaviour in the forced swim test, novelty suppressed feeding paradigm, and the sucrose splash test.

Conclusions:

These data show that ketamine can induce persistent stress resilience and, therefore, may be useful in protecting against stress-induced disorders.[1]

So a single dose of ketamine given prior to stress gave protection lasting for more than four weeks and was more effective than when given after stress. Christine Ann Denny, assistant professor at the Department of Psychiatry in Columbia University Medical Centre, is already considering trials for the use of prophylactic ketamine for people going into stressful situations (e.g. front-line soldiers and disaster relief workers).

A ketamine vaccine, an inoculation to improve our resilience in stressful situations—that would be truly exciting!

In summary let's review some of the elephants in the ketamine room. Ketamine works more quickly, more effectively, and with fewer side effects than our current treatments for treatment-resistant depression. Should it be our first-choice therapy in this situation?

The ketamine analogues currently being developed by pharmaceutical companies are unlikely to be more effective than ketamine, they will need time to be developed, there will be ongoing uncertainty concerning their long-term effects, and they will be vastly more expensive for both patients and society. Should we be waiting for them?

Ketamine works best for early episodes of depression. If used quickly as a first-line treatment, it has enormous potential to reduce the personal, social, and economic damage that arises from depressive illness. Should ketamine be used to treat a first episode of depression?

Ketamine has the potential to increase our resilience in stressful situations, and in the same way that we are inoculated against other diseases, it could be a successful prophylactic against pathological reactions to high-stress situations. Will it be suitable as a preventative medicine?

For every person who uses ketamine recreationally, there are a thousand who take it for good medical reasons. It is time to reclaim ketamine from the streets.

Future governments should both promote and subsidise the delivery of ketamine to those in need. There are great economic benefits associated with the rapid recovery seen with the use of low-dose ketamine. When we add to this reduced suicide rates, reduced personal and social disruption, improved efficiency at work, and massive savings in healthcare costs, ketamine truly has the potential to become the 'penicillin' of psychiatry.

References

1. R. A. Brachman, C. A. Denny, et al., 'Ketamine as a Prophylactic against Stress-Induced Depressive-Like Behaviour', *Biological Psychiatry* (4 May 2015). DOI: 10.1016/j.biopsych.2015.04.022.

Chapter 15

Summary: The Inconvenient Facts

Ketamine works for the majority of those who try it. It can significantly reduce suffering and, for some, completely relieve symptoms—all this with relatively few unwanted effects.

The short-term and long-term side effects are largely known and manageable.

On balance, the benefits hugely outweigh the risks, particularly when we include the personal, social, and economic risks of not treating severe chronic depression effectively. It can be safely taken at home in low dosage, giving many more sufferers the opportunity to try it for themselves.

Tolerance to the antidepressant effect is uncommon so any relapses can be treated quickly. This reduces a whole range of harms, including strained relationships, time away from work, and the use of harmful self-remedies, such as alcohol, gambling, and illicit drugs. Ketamine very rarely leads to dependence or addiction when used as recommended for medical reasons.

There are a number of alternative ways of giving ketamine and a range of possible venues for its use. Hospital treatment is suitable for acutely suicidal patients lacking supportive relationships and for those with physical problems requiring close observation and intensive management. There are specialised clinics for those needing higher doses of ketamine for treatment as possible side effects can be closely monitored and managed. They are also suitable settings when the risk of diversion or abuse is high as no takeaway doses would be given.

However, for the majority of patients, a general psychiatrist is best placed to make a thorough assessment, check out any physical health issues, and make a decision with the patient about the suitability of ketamine treatment. The low-dose sublingual treatment can be started in the office and then continued at home, with regular follow-up phone calls and appointments being made to check progress.

What is required, regardless of setting, is an accurate diagnosis and a thorough medical assessment which rules out other causes of depression. This would be followed by proper trials of proven remedies. Ketamine should always be given as part of a comprehensive treatment plan, including counselling on strategies for identifying stressors and managing them more effectively, thus reducing the risk of relapse. One of the most impressive effects of ketamine is that it allows people to be more open to change and, as their mood lifts, to be more able to restructure their lives.

We do not need to wait for the new alternatives which are being developed and patented and will be marketed to us no doubt at great expense to the public and private purse. There is no certainty that they will be as effective as ketamine, and there will still be the issue of unknown long-term side effects with these new products.

Some may be content to wait, but I am not, and none of my patients who were given the available facts had any hesitation in deciding to give it a try. As one said to me, 'Even a 10% improvement so that I have a bit more energy, shout at the kids a little less, and smile sometimes—that would make it worthwhile' (my patient, FC).

What is needed is a willing patient, a willing doctor, and an informed conversation about what is known and what is yet to be learned. Let the overzealous regulators, the fearmongers, and special-interest groups stand aside.

The inconvenient facts that low-dose ketamine can be both safely and effectively used to treat depression in a variety of settings, including a patient's own home, will be hard to accept for:

- those who say that ketamine does not work
- those who say that the dangers of addiction outweigh any possible benefit

- those who say that all patients should be treated under close supervision in hospitals
- those who fear a surge of ketamine-related harms if it becomes more frequently prescribed
- those who want to wait for new products to be developed, which will be unsullied by ketamine's reputation and unwanted effects
- those who want to wait until evermore clarifying research is available.

There are no magic bullets. This is not the holy grail, but ketamine is certainly a very useful addition to our current range of treatments. In my opinion, it is the most important advance I've seen in the treatment of patients suffering from depression in my 46 years as a doctor.

It is available now.

And in the end, as Edward F. Domino, would say, 'If in doubt, ask the patient.'

Well, when I did, one of my patients commented, 'It did not work for me, but I'm really glad I had the chance to try it. It gives me hope that something else will be along very soon.'

It is impossible to live without hope. Ketamine is many things to many people, but most of all, it's hope.

APPENDICES

Appendix 1

Patient Information Brochure

What is ketamine?

Ketamine is a medication that has been widely used as an anaesthetic agent since 1970 both in humans and in animals. In the last 18 years, it has been found helpful for people with pain conditions and, more recently, for people with psychiatric disorders.

How does it work?

Research has not yet determined completely how ketamine acts, but one finding is that there is a rapid regrowth of connections between brain neurones following treatment.

What does a trial of sublingual ketamine involve?

You will come into your doctor's rooms, and a very small dose of the drug will be given to you. The medicine is to be taken sublingually (that is to say, under the tongue). Please try not to swallow but hold the medicine under your tongue for three to four minutes until it is absorbed.

We would ask you to remain seated for an hour after the drug has been given as you may feel light-headed when you get up.

The drug starts working after about five minutes and will be mostly out of your system after an hour and a half, at which time you will be cleared to leave in the company of a friend or relative who will take you home.

What happens after the trial dose?

Your doctor will instruct you how to self-administer ketamine at home. The timing and dose levels will be explained. Your doctor will arrange follow-up appointments, emails and phone calls to adjust dosage and timing.

Benefits

Unfortunately, we cannot guarantee you will gain benefit from this treatment, but around 70% of people in clinical trials have reported improvement in psychiatric symptoms.

Alternatives

Your doctor will discuss alternatives with you in your consultation. These would include different medicines, counselling, and physical therapies. Every patient is unique, and therefore, specific alternatives cannot be given on an information leaflet as not all treatments are suitable for everyone.

What are the side effects?

You are advised not to drive or operate machinery for four hours after taking your medicine. Sleepiness may occur for a short period after taking the medicine. If this occurs, future doses can be taken at bedtime.

You may also experience a sensation that everything feels 'unreal' or 'far away'. This will only last for a short while and will soon disappear.

If you take too much ketamine or are very sensitive to its effects, you may go to sleep or have unusual dreams and hallucinations. We do not know a great deal about long-term problems that may occur using this medicine. Some studies suggest that there may be difficulties for some with memory loss or thought processing. There are also reports of effects on the liver and the bladder, but these are considered unlikely at the doses being used here. These problems seem to occur in some who take very high doses for extended periods for non-medical reasons. Reports of patients becoming dependent or addicted to ketamine when used as a medical treatment are very rare.

Ketamine is not currently licensed for use in psychiatric disorders or for chronic pain. There are many drugs that are not licensed for every condition, but they get used anyway because they work. It is quite often the case that a drug company will not apply for a licence for a drug for a particular condition or age group as the studies that they need to do may be too expensive or time consuming to be worth their while.

Although patients who take unlicensed drugs do so at their own risk, generally the risk is not great when measured against the possible benefits, and you and your doctor will make a considered judgement as to whether it is reasonable to use this treatment in your particular case.

What are patients normally taught to do?

You will be taught how to self-administer ketamine at home. Generally speaking, most people need to take it about two to three times a week to begin with, then the dosage and the time between doses are adjusted according to response. As there is the potential for ketamine to be misused it should be kept securely out of harm's way, and it would be wise not to discuss your use of it outside the family.

Further Information

Any questions arising from this leaflet should be raised with your doctor before signing your consent-for-treatment form.

Appendix 2

Consent to Treatment with Ketamine

Patient's name:
DOB:
Procedure: administration of sublingual ketamine

Doctor's Statement

In my opinion, there is no reason to doubt this patient's capacity to make this decision.

I have explained the treatment to the patient. In particular, I have described the intended benefits, including:

- reduction in feelings of depression, anxiety, and obsessive-compulsive symptoms
- reduced suicidal thoughts
- improved function.

I have also outlined significant, unavoidable, or frequently occurring risks, including short-term effects of dry mouth, nausea, dizziness, light-headedness, feelings of unreality, and rarely, hallucinations.

Long-term effects are unclear, but cognitive difficulties, bladder problems, and elevated liver enzymes have been reported in some with regular high-dose usage. Less than 1% of patients have problems with misuse of ketamine.

I have also discussed:

- that this currently is an off-label use of ketamine
- what the procedure involves, including financial costs
- any particular concerns of the patient
- the risks and benefits of alternative treatments, including no treatment.

I have provided the ketamine patient information leaflet.

Signed   Date

Name

Statement and Signature of Patient

You will be offered a copy of this form. You have the right to change your mind at any time, including after you have signed this form.

I have read the Patient Information Leaflet.

I understand the information that I have been given about the treatment described on this form.

I agree to the course of treatment described on this form.

Patient's signature:

Date:

Appendix 3

Ketamine Prescriptions

Throughout the world there are different regulations governing the use of ketamine. In Australia, ketamine is currently designated as an S8 medication. The RANZCP in December of 2017 updated their memorandum on the use of ketamine for treatment-resistant depression, effectively supporting its use outside of hospitals and clinical trials, subject to certain conditions. However, each state has its own regulations governing prescribing and some of the states e.g Tasmania have been extremely slow in updating their regulations to reflect the RANZCP's new position.

In Australia ketamine is currently not covered by the PBS and it is prescribed using standard script forms. Some of the prescription costs may be refundable to those with private health coverage.

Sublingual ketamine may administered as a liquid, a wafer, or in lozenge form, all with different strengths. It is wise to work with one pharmacy where possible and to discuss with them availability, practicality and costs.

1. Herewith is a sample prescription for the 10 mg/ml oral solution:

    Rx:
    Ketamine hydrochloride oral solution 10 mg/ml.
    Take 1–3 ml (one to three millilitres) sublingually every second day.

Mitte:
20 ml (twenty millilitres) of 10 mg/ml oral solution and two repeats.
Minimum dispensing interval 7 days.

2. Herewith is a sample prescription for the 100 mg/ml oral
   solution:

Rx:
Ketamine hydrochloride oral solution 100 mg/ml.
Take 0.5–1.0 ml (point five to one millilitres) sublingually every
   two to seven days.

Mitte:
5 ml (5 millilitres) of the 100 mg/ml oral solution and two repeats.
Minimum dispensing interval 10 days.

Appendix 4

Ketamine Treatment Schedule

Check diagnosis and alternative options; check that current treatments are compatible.

Assess the following relative contraindications:

- allergy to ketamine
- unstable cardiovascular illness
- severe liver impairment
- severe kidney/bladder disease
- current addiction to ketamine
- current psychotic illness
- closed angle glaucoma
- pregnancy.

The following tests may be helpful (if indicated):

- urine dipstick, midstream urine MSU, renal function, liver function
- blood pressure (BP) and pulse rate
- body mass index (BMI), electrocardiogram (ECG), C-reactive protein (CRP).

On treatment day do the following:

- Check that you have a benzodiazepine and an antihypertensive agent available and a clear plan if there are any untoward responses (e.g. allergic reactions).
- Document visual analogue scale readings.
- Discuss the ketamine information leaflet.
- Sign the ketamine treatment form.
- Establish basal BP and pulse rate.

During treatment do the following:

- Monitor BP and pulse rate.
- Assess for side effects.
- Have a 60-to-90-minute observation period.
- Ensure safe transport is available.

The following are required during the follow-up period:

- phone calls, email contact, and visits as practicable
- patients to record daily VAS recordings
- doses every two days initially, then according to response
- adjustments to dosage and time between doses according to response and side effects.

Index

Made in the USA
Coppell, TX
10 October 2022